Profiles
of Nurse
Healers

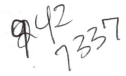

Profile of Nurse Healers

Lynn Keegan, RN, PhD, HNC, FAAN
Associate Professor, University of Texas
Health Science Center at San Antonio
School of Nursing
Co-Director, Bodymind Systems
Temple, Texas

Barbara Montgomery Dossey, RN, MS, HNC, FAAN
Director, Holistic Nursing Consultants
Sante Fè, New Mexico
Co-Director, Bodymind Systems
Temple, Texas

Delmar Publishers

I(T)P®

an International Thomson Publishing Company

Albany • Bonn • Boston • Cincinnati • Detroit • London
Madrid • Melbourne • Mexico City • New York • Pacific Grove
Paris • San Francisco • Singapore • Tokyo • Toronto • Washington

NOTICE TO THE READER

Publisher does not warrant or guarantee any of the products described herein or perform any independent analysis in connection with any of the product information contained herein. Publisher does not assume, and expressly disclaims, any obligation to obtain and include information other than that provided to it by the manufacturer.

The reader is expressly warned to consider and adopt all safety precautions that might be indicated by the activities described herein and to avoid all potential hazards. By following the instructions contained herein, the reader willingly assumes all risks in connection with such instructions.

The publisher makes no representations or warranties of any kind, including but not limited to, the warranties of fitness for particular purpose or merchantability, nor are any such representations implied with respect to the material set forth herein, and the publisher takes no responsibility with respect to such material. The publisher shall not be liable for any special, consequential, or exemplary damages resulting, in whole or in part, from the readers' use of, or reliance upon, this material.

Sci
RT
34
K44
1998

Delmar Staff
Publisher: William Brottmiller
Acquisitions Editor: Greg Vis
Assistant Editor: Hilary Schrauf
Production Editor: Marah Bellegarde

COPYRIGHT © 1998
By Delmar Publishers
a division of International Thomson Publishing
The ITP logo is a trademark under license.

Printed in the United States of America

For more information, contact:

Delmar Publishers
3 Columbia Circle, Box 15015
Albany, New York 12212-5015

International Thomson Publishing - Europe
Berkshire House 168-173
High Holborn
London, WC1V7AA
England

Thomas Nelson Australia
102 Dodds Street
South Melbourne, 3205
Victoria, Australia

Nelson Canada
1120 Birchmont Road
Scarborough, Ontario
Canada, M1K 5G4

International Thomson Editores
Campos Eliseos 385, Piso 7
Col Polanco
11560 Mexico DF Mexico

International Thomson Publishing GmbH
Königswinterer Strasse 418
53227 Bonn
Germany

International Thomson Publishing Asia
221 Henderson Road
#05-10 Henderson Building
Singapore 0315

International Thomson Publishing - Japan
Hirakawacho Kyowa Building, 3F
2-2-1 Hirakawacho
Chiyoda-ku, Tokyo 102
Japan

1 2 3 4 5 6 7 8 9 10 XXX 03 02 01 00 99 98 97

Library of Congress Cataloging-in-Publication Data

Keegan, Lynn.
    Profiles of nurse healers / Lynn Keegan, Barbara Montgomery Dossey.
        p. cm. — (Nurse as healer series)
    Includes bibliographical references and index.
    ISBN 0-8273-7958-7
    1. Nurses—Biography. 2. Holistic nursing. 3. Healing.
I. Dossey, Barbara Montgomery. II. Title. III. Series
RT34.K44 1997
610.73'092'2—dc21
[B]

97–7960
CIP

DEDICATION

To our Colleagues in Nursing:
Who are exploring new meanings of healing in
their work
Who are facilitating healing in their own lives
Who are recognizing their role as nurse healers

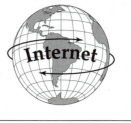

INTRODUCTION TO NURSE AS HEALER SERIES

LYNN KEEGAN, RN, PhD, HNC, FAAN, Series Editor
*Associate Professor, School of Nursing,
University of Texas Health Science Center at San Antonio
and Director of Bodymind Systems, Temple, TX*

To nurse means to care for or to nurture with compassion. Most nurses begin their formal education with this ideal. Many nurses retain this orientation after graduation, and some manage their entire careers under this guiding principle of caring. Many of us, however, tend to forget this ideal in the hectic pace of our professional and personal lives. We may become discouraged and feel a sense of burnout.

Throughout the past decade I have spoken at many conferences with thousands of nurses. Their experience of frustration and failure is quite common. These nurses feel themselves spread as pawns across a health care system too large to control or understand. In part, this may be because they have forgotten their true roles as nurse-healers.

When individuals redirect their personal vision and empower themselves, an entire pattern may begin to change. And so it is now with the nursing profession. Most of us conceptualize nursing as much more than a vocation. We are greater than our individual roles as scientist, specialists, or care deliverers. We currently search for a name to put on our new conception of the empowered nurse. The recently introduced term nurse healer aptly describes the qualities of an increasing number of clinicians, educators, administrators, and nurse practitioners. Today all nurses are awakening to the realization that they have the potential for healing.

It is my feeling that most nurses, when awakened and guided to develop their own healing potential, will function both as nurses and healers. Thus, the concept of nurse as healer is born. When nurses realize they have the ability to evoke others' healing, as well as care for them, a shift of consciousness begins to occur. As individual awareness and changes in skill building occur, a collective understanding of this new concept emerges. This knowledge, along with a shift in attitudes and new kinds of behavior, allows empowered nurses to renew themselves in an expanded role. The Nurse As Healer Series is born out of the belief that nurses are ready to embrace guidance that inspires them in their journeys of empowerment. Each book in the series may stand alone or be used in complementary fashion with other books. I hope and believe that information herein will strengthen you both personally and professionally, and provide you with the help and confidence to embark upon the path of nurse healer.

Titles in the Nurse As Healer Series:

Awareness in Healing

Creative Imagery in Nursing

Energetic Approaches to Emotional Healing

Healing Addictions: The Vulnerability Model of Recovery

Healing the Dying

Healing and the Grief Process

Healing Life's Crises: A Guide for Nurses

Healing Meditation

Healing Nutrition

Healing Touch: A Resource for Health Care Professionals

The Nurse as Healer

The Nurse's Meditative Journal

C O N T E N T S

P R E F A C E

Nurse healers can be found in all areas of nursing. They live and work among us as colleagues, clinicians, educators, researchers, or are our personal practitioners. Unfortunately, the current situation is that nurse healers usually are unseen because the profession is still developing the criteria and parameters in which to recognize them. When we read or hear about healing journeys of nurse healers, they help us to develop insight of how to recognize and honor their work and vision. They also inspire us to strive for new ways of living and practicing the art and science of nursing.

This book is divided into four parts. Part 1 develops the role of nurse healers. Some of these areas are a holistic foundation, relationship-centered care, personal meanings in lived experiences, concepts of health-wellness-disease-illness, and integrating alternative/complementary therapies in various practice environments.

Part 2 explores the qualities of a nurse healer. The topics discussed are the caring-healing environment, nurse as healer, healing versus curing, the mind-body dilemma, the human spirit in healing, creating healing environments, patterns of knowing and unknowing, presence, the art of guiding, real versus pseudo-listening, and our relationships with others.

Part 3 presents nurse healer profiles and their healing journeys. The nurses featured in Part 3 are individuals who accepted an invitation to share their story in this book. The nurse healers presented represented a cross section of practicing professional nurses. They are in independent practice, education, acute care, chronic and long-term care, and administration. These nurse healers have made significant contributions at local and regional levels, and many are recognized as national leaders.

The nurse healers profiled were asked to write a brief biography including a statement about their origin, the journey they followed to become nurse healers, and to then conclude with a statement of advice to those who will model and join them in the best of contemporary nursing practice.

The essays are in the nurse healers' own words. As you read these stories, notice the similarities and differences among them and between them, and look for the themes inherent in most of them. You will find that for many the path they trod was not easy. There were peaks and valleys, obstacles, and challenges to overcome. Most tell about their personal wounding and healing into empowerment when they followed their vision for holistic nursing and holistic living.

In Part 4 strategies are presented to assist us in our personal healing journey. Featured topics include how to integrate healing rituals in daily living and clinical practice, mindfulness practice, journaling, how to explore creativity, sharing our healing stories, and brown bag lunch sessions.

Our book is intended for students, clinicians, educators, and researchers who desire to expand their knowledge of holism, healing, and spirituality. These profiles of nurse healers will challenge nurses to explore their inward journey toward self-transformation and to identify their growing capacity for change and healing. This effort creates the synergy and the rebirth of a compassionate power to heal ourselves and to facilitate healing within others.

The radical changes that are occurring in the profession of nursing and in health care reform are very dynamic. Always the rule in health care, change provides us with a greater opportunity to integrate caring and healing into our work, our research, and our lives.

This inner healing allows us to return to our roots of nursing where healer and healing were understood. If we are to capture our essence and emerge as true nurse healers on the doorsteps of the twenty-first century, we must unite and share our personal healing journeys and weave a larger healing tapestry about the art and science in our work and lives.

What image can you create and then hold of what and how you want your life and your role as a nurse healer to be at the turn of the century? What is captured in your mission statement about your personal and professional vision? As we further expand our mission statement and envision holism in our profession and lives, then we are better able to bring it into being. Best wishes in your healing journey.

Lynn Keegan
Barbara M. Dossey

A C K N O W L E D G E M E N T S

We celebrate with our colleagues in nursing as we explore new meanings of healing in our life and work. We acknowledge what we have done well, and we anticipate what we must do better. Our book flows out of the larger questions that have been raised for us in the health or illness of clients/patients and their families/significant others, our families, and the professional communities with whom we live and play.

Special thanks are due to Greg Vis, sponsoring editor at Delmar Publishers, Inc. who helped us keep our goals in sight and believed in our project; to Hilary Schrauf for handling the editorial details; to Marah Bellegarde for logo, book design, and production details; and to TDB Publishing Services

Most of all, for their understanding, encouragement, and love in seeing us through one more book, we thank our families—Gerald, Catherine, and Genevieve Keegan; and Larry Dossey.

I N T R O D U C T I O N

SHARING OUR HEALING JOURNEYS

In this book we will explore the journey towards wholeness in many ways, but first we would like to share with you how we got together and how each of us began our personal journey. We first met through the American Holistic Nurses' Association (AHNA) in 1981. Since that time we have been actively involved within the organization. We have also collaborated on many projects, and continue to be committed to the discipline of holistic nursing practice and its future developments. We each have had specific life events and clinical experiences that helped us to become more involved in caring and healing practices. We hope that our stories awaken your interest for all those that follow in this book.

LYNN KEEGAN, RN, PhD, HNC, FAAN

I knew I was going to be a nurse when I was fifteen years old. The decision came after caring for my mother following surgery. My mother was admitted for ligation and removal of varicose veins of both legs following the birth of four children and years on her feet. From my young perspective, and indeed it was in those days, the surgery seemed to be a complicated and difficult procedure and necessitated that my mother be taken from our home to the big medical center in Galveston, a day's drive away. I recall missing school and staying overnight to care for my mother in the large, open, surgical ward. She, and other postoperative women were nauseated and vomiting following the anesthesia of the day and moaning and crying due to their pain. I recall rushing from woman to woman to help them hold their metal emesis basin as they wretched and vomited, trying my best to comfort them in their sickness and pain. I undertook, in the only way I knew how, to help the busy night nurse who kept general unit control from her desk at one side of the ward and dispensed medications from the metal shelf on the wall behind her desk. Although too busy to do all that was needed with the patients, she was kind and seemed to have an air of control in her long, white, starched uniform. The prolonged, dark night and the women's needs seemed to go on forever. I recall thinking that now I knew exactly what I wanted to do, and that was to prepare myself to help alleviate the suffering of the sick.

The first person I told about my decision, the school nurse, seemed to think my goal was a good one. She encouraged me to become a member of the future nurses' club at school and helped me enroll at the local hospital's girls volunteer, Candy Stripe program. Here, on Saturday mornings, I delivered newspapers, mail, and books and visited with bed-bound patients. Since this was in the late 1950s, patients were still considered convalescent and most were on bedrest regimes.

At age sixteen, with a year of Saturday morning hospital experience under my belt, I was convinced my decision was right, I should become a nurse, and if I was to do it, I would get the best possible preparation. My role model, the high school nurse, only knew about diploma programs, but with the help of the county librarian, I discovered there were other paths. I reached out to the few baccalaureate programs in the country and began systematic correspondence to plan my academic career. With the aid of scholarships and loans and by working my way through school, I graduated from Cornell University, New York Hospital School of Nursing, a five-year baccalaureate degree program, in the mid 1960s.

In my early work experiences in acute care settings I focused on meeting the multifaceted physical needs of sick people while attending to the yet-to-be-defined emotional, mental, and spiritual needs that they also exhibited. It was during graduate school study for my master's degree in the late 1960s at a Seventh Day Adventist religious institution in California, Loma Linda University, that the consideration of a holistic approach was first brought to light. Here, spiritual, emotional, nutritional, and other components were considered in both the etiology and treatment of the patient.

Following graduation, I practiced from this broadened perspective in an acute care setting one more year prior to beginning to teach. I began academia back on the east coast and returned to the dominant theme of the day—a secular, pathophysiologic approach to care. It was some years later after moving to still another state and being assigned to teach in the graduate program that my return to holism was renewed and solidified. While an Assistant Professor at Texas Women's University, I was able to both teach and incorporate aspects of holistic nursing into all my class offerings. It was thrilling to be a part of personally living well and getting to share and incorporate that experience with students. It was also during this time that I became involved with the newly emerging American Holistic Nurses' Association, focused my research dissertation on holistic principles, and completed my doctoral studies.

During the mid 1980s I left traditional practice and opened a Wellness Center. It was here, while attending clients who were not physically ill, but who sought relief of stress symptoms, that I had the time and opportunity to work most closely with a holistic approach. During hour-long sessions, clients had the opportunity to trace back to their past as they considered future plans. Here they uncovered both physical and behavioral life style patterns and then could see how these patterns contributed to their current state of distress. Together we worked from a holistic perspective to plan for repatterning their lives for more healthy responses. In that work I used relaxation and imagery, biofeedback, touch therapies, nutritional and exercise counseling, and other modalities and nursing interventions to guide and assist these clients toward self-healing. It was in that practice that I firmly witnessed each individual's potential for awakening, the importance of guidance from a professional, and the ability of individuals to heal themselves.

For the past decade my life has been focused in academics, consultation, and authorship with the purpose of linking holism to everything I do. Today I teach university graduate classes and blend holism into all my teaching and research projects and expand upon these concepts in my consulting and authoring work. Another primary focus is to keep my nuclear family strong and unified while at the same time bringing a loving intention to the extended family that we all share.

Through active participation on national committies within several professional organizations, I have opportunities to meet and work in partnership with other holistic practitioners. Each of these connections builds upon the previous one to add layers of learning and satisfaction. In turn, the encounters with each individual and group relationship open new doors and, in walking through, I continually discover joy and new ways of being.

BARBARA MONTGOMERY DOSSEY, RN, MS, HNC, FAAN

Born in Little Rock, Arkansas, I was accompanied into this world by my fraternal twin brother; three years later our dear sister came along. I was blessed to be part of a close family where I learned about unconditional love.

I gave no thought to a professional career until my sophomore year in high school. My older cousin was a nursing supervisor and a very wise woman. Her stories about nursing and the hospital always fascinated me. On one visit to see my relatives, my uncle was the first to suggest the value of a nursing career. Later, his other two daughters also became nurses. The seed was planted, and several weeks later when my sophomore counselor asked me what I wanted to study in college, I responded nursing. Thus began my journey.

After thirty-three years of being in the world of health care, the challenge for me with patients, their families, and my colleagues has been to teach rituals that integrate a person's belief systems and their innate healing ability with modern technology. Much of my professional career has been spent with patients and their families as they face cardiovascular disease and critical illness.

There have been many technologic breakthroughs in cardiovascular disease such as pacemakers, coronary artery bypass surgery, heart assist devices, and procedures and medications to open up and clean out coronary arteries. However, the cause and cure for many cardiovascular problems still have not been discovered. So we are painfully aware that the sophisticated technology and medications really do not provide all the answers in preventing, stabilizing, and reversing cardiovascular illness. We are also aware that the current Western medical model does not explain the psychologic, social, or spiritual causes of the disease. Why then is the medical model still falling short of predicted criteria? Could it be that after all these centuries we now realize that the biomedical model can never provide us with complete answers in treating heart disease, cancer, and other major illnesses. For it has never taken into account the profound devastating affects or the enormous healing effects of a person's mind and spirit on the body. We are at a time in history where we must transform our health care system from a disease management industry to a healing system.

I entered cardiovascular and critical care nursing in the early sixties at a time when the thoughts, emotions, and beliefs of the patients and families were more valued by physicians and nurses who practiced an authentic kind of healing. As technology increased so did impersonal interactions, specialization, and a focus on curing of symptoms. When a patient got well, it was attributed to the machines and the potent medications. The meaning of illness and its place and purpose in a person's life became anachronistic.

Early in my career, I became aware of the power of a person's belief systems. My first head nurse taught me the importance of what it meant to serve another in the midst of the fast-paced, technologic, critical care environment. She emphasized the nurse's presence, the quality of being present with a person without doing anything. She told me to listen with my heart and to feel as much as possible what a patient believed to be true. As I have listened to the rich tapestry of patients' life stories, I have realized that the meanings that they gave their lives and the healing rituals that they incorporated, for the most part, directed how they would heal, almost without regard to medical technology or treatments used.

In the late sixties I began my own personal journey of learning self-regulation strategies due primarily to a medical condition, dendritic keratitis (herpes simplex of the cornea). Whenever I was under stress, it would flare up and over a seven-year period, I developed severe scar formation on my right cornea. By the end of 1974, I had gone a full year without a flare up which at the time was the criteria for a corneal transplant. About six weeks after my transplant, I had an acute rejection that was managed by an injection of steroid into my eye. An eyelid stretcher was placed around my right eye to keep my eye open while receiving the injection. Later as I reflected on the anxiety I felt with that injection, I was more attune to the anxiety and fear of the patients I was caring for in the critical care unit. The anxiety of seeing the needle coming toward my eye and the helplessness I felt never left my consciousness. It made me aware of being more present with my patients before I poked, suctioned, etc. during all the procedures and treatments. Around this time I began to read about psychophysiologic stress, and became attuned to the fact that I did not know how to consistently manage my own stress levels. It was clear to me that one aspect of my recurrent eye condition was related to stress as was my rejection process. I seriously pursued biofeedback, relaxation, imagery, how to play more, and how to take personal time to do nothing. As I integrated new life style behaviors, my clinical practice also began to change. It became very obvious to me that the self-regulation strategies that I was using in my own life could also be taught to patients and incorporated in the critical care unit as well as in all areas of nursing. In the seventies, exciting research on interactions of beliefs and emotions on physiology and healing appeared in leading professional journals. I now had scientific validation of what I had witnessed since the beginning of my career.

As I learned more about self-regulation skills and integrated them into my own life, my professional practice was enhanced. I began to teach these same self-regulation skills to patients in the critical care unit and in cardiac rehabilitation programs. It was thrilling to participate with patients and their families as they shared their stories and healing rituals with each other and learned how to alter their own biochemistry and decrease their fear and anxiety. For example, patients in significant pain could learn how to distract themselves from the pain with relaxation and imagery exercises; a patient with minimal blood flow to his severely injured left leg used relaxation and imagery skills to increase blood flow to his injured leg and avoided amputation. With a change in attitude and being empowered, these patients' body chemicals and inner healing resources worked toward their recovery rather than to impede their healing. This repeated experience with many patients and their families allowed me to deeply understand the importance of rituals and the rich tapestry of the interconnectedness of body-mind-spirit.

Currently, teaching and writing in the areas of self-regulation and healing is my focus. Assisting people to identify their belief systems, their inner world of images, and to find their own pathways to wellness with personal rituals continues to be a healing journey. The joy of facilitating this process deepens my rich experiences as I continue to weave my own caring-healing journey with my family, friends, and colleagues.

CONTRIBUTORS

Jean Sayre-Adams, RN, MA
Director, Didsbury Trust
Bath, England

Veda L. Andrus, RN, EdD, HNC
Program Director, AHNA
   Certificate Program in Holistic
   Nursing
Whately, Massachusetts

**Irene Wade Belcher, RN, MS,
   CNS**
Senior Editor, AHNA Beginnings
   Newsletter
Tucker, Georgia

**Rita Benor, RGN, RM, RNT,
   RHV, Cert Ed. Couns. Cert,
   M. BAFATT**
Psychotherapist, Autogenic
   Training Therapist, Bach
   Flower Practitioner, Lecturer
   in Complementary
   Therapies/Medicine
Rockville, Maryland

**Wailua Brandman, RN, MSN,
   CS, NP**
Instructor of Nursing, Advanced
   Practice Program, University
   of Hawaii at Manoa
Manoa, Hawaii

**Ernestina Handy Briones, RN,
   PhD**
Nursing Administrator, Valley
   Baptist Medical Center
Harlingen, Texas

**Margaret A. Burkhart, RN,
   PhD, CS**
Associate Professor, School of
   Nursing, Robert C. Byrd
   Health Science Center of
   West Virginia University
Charleston, West Virginia

**Susan B. Collins, RN, MS,
   FNP, HNC**
Clinical Director, North
   Country Community
   Health Center
Flagstaff, Arizona

**Anne L. Day, RN, MA, PNP,
   CMT, CHTP/I**
National Instructor of Healing
   Touch, Journaling and
   Presence, Red Rock Com-
   munity College Holistic Nurs-
   ing Instructor, Massage,
   Healing Touch, and
   Wellness Counseling
   Practitioner, Founder and
   Owner of Healing Touch
   Hawaii
Golden, Colorado

**Helen Lorraine Erickson, RN,
   PhD, HNC, FAAN**
Professor, School of Nursing,
   University of Texas
   at Austin
Austin, Texas

Martha Fortune, RN, MS
Nurse Consultant, Community
   Nursing Organization,
   Visiting Nurse Association
   of New York
New York, New York

Mary J. Frost, RN, MS, CHTP/I
Co-founder & Educational
   Director, Total Health, Inc.,
   Holistic Nursing Associates
   and Consultants
Covington, Louisiana

Cathie E. Guzzetta, RN, PhD, FAAN
Director, Holistic Nursing
  Consultants, Nursing Research
  Consultant, Parkland
  Memorial Hospital and
  Children's Medical Center
  of Dallas
Dallas, Texas

Merla R. Hoffman, RN, MSN, HNC, CHTP/I
Holistic Nursing Consultant and
  Educator
Colorado Springs, Colorado

Dorothea Hover-Kramer, RN, EdD, CHTP/I
Licensed Clinical Psychologist
  and Director Behavioral
  Health Consultants
Poway, California

Ruth L. Johnson, RN, PhD
Co-founder and Director,
  HAPPEN
Black Mountain, North Carolina

Rita L Kluny, RN, BSN, CHTP/I
Neonatal and Pediatric Critical
  Care Nurse
New Orleans, Louisana

JoEllen Koerner, RN, PhD, FAAN
Senior Vice President of Patient
  Services, Sioux Valley
  Hospital
Sioux Falls, South Dakota

Susan Luck, RN, MA
HIV Patient Coordinator, Health
  Educator, Stratogen Health of
  Miami Beach
Miami Beach, Florida

Sandra Lutz, RN, MS, CFNP, CHTP/I
PRN Planned Parenthood,
  Private Practice, Healing
  Touch Instructor
Perkins, Illinois

Maggie McKivergin, RN, MS
Life Coach/Consultant
Columbus, Ohio

Susan Morales, RN, MSN, CHTP/I
Director, Healing Touch Canada,
  Inc., President, Canadian
  Healing Touch Foundation
Toronto, Ontario, Canada

Melodie Olson, RN, PhD
Associate Professor, College of
  Nursing, Medical University
  of South Carolina
Charleston, South Carolina

Glenda Pitts, RN, MSN, HNC
Private Practice
Louisville, Kentucky

Janet Quinn, RN, PhD, FAAN
Associate Professor and Senior
  Scholar, Center for Human
  Caring, School of Nursing,
  University of Colorado Health
  Sciences Center
Denver, Colorado

Lynn Rew, RN, EdD, C, HNC, FAAN
Associate Professor, School of
  Nursing, The University
  of Texas at Austin, Editor,
  Journal of Holistic Nursing
Austin, Texas

Sharon Scandrett-Hibdon, RN, PhD, FNP, CHTP/I
Private Practice, Educator
Aubrey, Texas

Eleanor Ann Schuster, RN, DNSc
Associate Professor, College of
  Nursing, Florida Atlantic
  University
Boca Raton, Florida

**Karilee Halo Shames, RN, PhD,
  HNC**
Director, Nurse Empowerment
  Workshops and Services,
  Private Practice
Mill Valley, California

Jill Strawn, RN, MSN, CS
Doctoral Candidate, Columbia
  University, New York, Adjunct
  Faculty, School of Nursing,
  College of New Rochelle,
New Rochelle, New York

Donna Taliaferro, RN, PhD, CNS
Assistant Professor, School of
  Nursing, University of Texas
  Health Science Center
  at San Antonio
San Antonio, Texas

Marilee Tolen, RN, HNC, CHTP/I
CEO/President, Corporate Wellness
  Consultants, Inc.
Cherry Hill, New Jersey

**Jean Marie Umlor, RSM, RN, MNA,
  HNC**
Coordinator of Holistic Clinical
  Practice, Mercy Health Services
  North
Cadillac/Grayling, Michigan

**Joan Vitello-Cicciu, RN, MSN,
  CCRN, CS, FAAN**
Acting Nurse Manager Emergency
  Department, Boston Medical
  Center, East Newton Campus
Boston, Massachusetts

**Marsha Jelonek Walker, RN, MSN,
  RMT**
Holistic Nurse Educator, Registered
  Massage Therapist
Austin, Texas

**Carol Wells-Federman, RN, MS,
  MEd, CS**
Co-Director, Chronic Pain Clinic
  Division of Behavioral Medicine,
  Beth Israel Deaconess Medical
  Center, Associate in Medicine,
  Harvard Medical School
Boston, Massachusetts

Bonnie Wesorick, RN, MS
Director, Clinical Practice Model
  (CPM) Resource Center,
  Butterworth Hospital
Grand Rapids, Michigan

**Wendy Wetzel, RN, MSN, FNP,
  HNC**
Nurse Practitioner, A Woman's Place
Flagstaff, Arizona

Patty Wooten, RN, BSN, CCRN
Nurse Humorist
Davis, California

Anneke Young, RN, BSN, CNAT
Director, Wholistic Nursing School,
  New Center College, Associate
  Director, Wholistic Health Center,
  New Center College
Syosset, New York

Part

1 THE ROLE OF NURSE HEALERS

1

THE ROLE
OF
NURSE HEALERS

INTRODUCTION

Nurse healers have been influential in the development of the discipline of holistic nursing. The nurses who have contributed to this development are aware of the importance of developing and integrating a holistic perspective in all aspects of their personal and professional lives. A nurse healer is one who facilitates another person's growth toward wholeness—body, mind, spirit—or who assists one with recovery from illness or with transition to peaceful death (Dossey, 1995a; Keegan, 1994).

NURSE HEALERS' HOLISTIC FOUNDATIONS

Over the last twenty-five years, medicine has been driven by biotechnology when confronting disease, trauma, and complications. This has had a direct impact on the nursing profession and on client/patient care. At present the health care system still operates from a scientific paradigm that separates an individual into a biologic, psychologic, sociologic, and spiritual being. The health care system is faced with challenges to operate from a holistic perspective rather than from the limitations of a traditional or allopathic model. Allopathy is the method of combating disease with techniques that produce effects different from those produced by the disease.

Nurse healers are dynamic individuals who recognize the changes needed to reform a biotechnology driven health care system to become a relationship-centered care driven healing system. They pursue personal, clinical, educational, and research approaches to address these complex interconnected processes so that they can provide relationship-centered care. They take action to enhance caring and healing at personal levels and in various professional levels of clinical practice and healthcare reform.

Nurse healers understand that human beings must be viewed from a holistic perspective. They practice relationship-centered care and integrate the strategies necessary to implement relationship-centered caring. As part of their overall vision nurse healers have to be part of a health care system that is driven by the needs of clients/patients and significant others where they make optimal contributions. Nurse healers recognize holistic nursing as the most complete way to conceptualize and practice professional nursing. The American Holistic Nurses' Association working description of holistic nursing is shown in Figure 1-1 (American Holistic Nurses' Association, 1994a).

Nurse healers utilize concepts of holistic nursing that are based on broad and eclectic academic principles. They are guided by the American Holistic Nurses' Association Standards of Holistic Nursing Practice as shown in Figure 1-2 (American Holistic Nurses'

DESCRIPTION OF HOLISTIC NURSING

Holistic nursing embraces all nursing practice which has healing the whole person as its goal. Holistic nursing recognizes that there are two views regarding holism: that holism involves studying and understanding the interrelationships of the bio-psycho-social-spiritual dimensions of the person, recognizing that the whole is greater than the sum of its parts; and that holism involves understanding the individual as an integrated whole interacting with and being acted upon by both internal and external environments. Holistic nursing accepts both views, believing that the goals of nursing can be achieved within either framework

Holistic practice draws on nursing knowledge, theories, expertise, and intuition to guide nurses in becoming therapeutic partners with clients in strengthening the clients' responses to facilitate the healing process and achieve wholeness.

Practicing holistic nursing requires nurses to integrate self-care in their own lives. Self-responsibility leads the nurse to a greater awareness of the interconnectedness of all individuals and their relationships to the human and global community, and permits nurses to use this awareness to facilitate healing.

Source: Copyright © American Holistic Nurses' Association, January 1994.

FIGURE 1-1 *Description of Holistic Nursing*

CORE VALUES ADDRESSED IN HOLISTIC NURSING PRACTICE

PART I: DISCIPLINE OF HOLISTIC NURSING PRACTICE

Core Value I.   Holistic Philosphy
Core Value II.   Holistic Foundation
Core Value III.   Holistic Ethics
Core Value IV.   Holistic Nursing Theories
Core Value V.   Holistic Nursing and Related Research
Core Value VI.   Holistic Nursing Process

PART II: CARING FOR THE WHOLE CLIENT
                AND SIGNIFICANT OTHERS

Core Value VII.   Meaning and Wholeness
Core Value VIII.   Client Self-Care
Core Value IX.   Health Promotion

Source: Based on a working document of the American Holistic Nurses' Association. Copyright © March, 1997, Revised. The American Holistic Nurses' Association, 4101 Lake Boone Trail, Suite 201, Raleigh, NC 27607. Phone 1-800-278-AHNA Fax (919) 787-4916. Used with permission.

FIGURE 1-2 *Core values addressed in Holistic Nursing Practice*

Association, 1997b, Revised). These standards incorporate the use of nursing and related theory and research-based practice that assist nurse healers with ways to analyze client/patient outcomes and to evaluate client/patient care. This assists them with the necessary steps to address continuous quality improvement. Nurse healers incorporate a sensitive balance between the art and science, and analytic and intuitive skills that enhance the interconnectedness of body, mind, and spirit. They consider the integrated whole to understand the person or situation. Nurse healers are aware that these concepts are essential in order to participate in the dynamics strategies necessary to implement relationship-center care.

RELATIONSHIP-CENTERED CARE

Nurse healers now and in the future will become more engaged in relationship-centered care. The Pew Health Professions Commission on Health Professions Education has described the three components of relationship-centered care as follows: client/-patient-practitioner relationship, community-practitioner relationship, and practitioner-practitioner relationship (Tresolini, 1994). Each of these interrelated relationships is essential within a reformed system of health care. Each of the components involves a unique set of tasks and responsibilities that addresses four areas: self-awareness, knowledge, values, and skills. As nurse healers participate in the dynamics within these three components of relationship-centered care, they will demonstrate a more integrated and comprehensive view of the work they do and the way they live their lives. As role models they are creating the necessary changes in health care delivery and health care reform as well as having a direct and positive impact on their communities.

Client/Patient-Practitioner Relationship

Nurse healers are evolving new levels of client/patient healing encounters. In a client/patient-practitioner relationship, the practitioner within this relationship collects data about the patient's symptoms and individual needs as well as to incorporate the comprehensive biotechnological care. Active collaboration with the client/patient and the family in the decision-making process and promoting health and preventing stress/illness within the family are also part of the relationship. It involves reflecting on skills and practice of increasing self-awareness of caring, healing, values, ethics, and ways to enhance and preserve the dignity and integrity of the client/patient and the family. It also involves active listening and communicating effectively. A nurse healer seeks to reduce the power inequalities with regard to race, sex, education, occupation, and socioeconomic status.

To work effectively within the client/patient-practitioner relationships the practitioner must develop knowledge, skills, and values in four areas as summarized in Table 1-1: self-awareness; the client/patient's experience of health and illness; developing and maintaining relationships with client/patients; and communicating clearly and effectively (Tresoloni, 1994).

Community-Practitioner Relationship

Nurse healers are developing increased awareness in the complexity and range of relationships and cultural diversity of individuals. The client/patient and his or her family and significant others simultaneously belong to many types of communities such as the hospital community, immediate family, relatives, friends, co-workers, neighborhoods, religious and community organizations, and so

TABLE 1-1 *Health Professions Education and Relationship-Centered Care Patient-Practitioner Relationship: Areas of Knowledge, Skills and Values. Courtesy of PEW Health Professions Commission at the Center for the Health Professions, University of California, San Francisco, California.*

AREA	KNOWLEDGE	SKILLS	VALUES
Self-awareness	Knowledge of self Understanding self as a resource to others	Reflect on self and work	Importance of self-awareness, self-care, self-growth
Patient experience of health and illness	Role of family, culture, community in development Multiple components of health Multiple threats and contributors to health as dimensions of one reality	Recognize patient's life story and its meaning View health and illness as part of human development	Appreciation of the patient as a whole person Appreciation of the patient's life story and the meaning of the health-illness condition
Developing and maintaining caring relationships	Understanding of threats to the integrity of the relationship (e.g. power inequalities) Understanding of potential for conflict and abuse	Attend fully to the patient Accept and respond to distress in patient and self Respond to moral and ethical challenges Facilitate hope, trust, and faith	Respect for patient's dignity, uniqueness, and integrity (mind-body-spirit unity) Respect for self-determination Respect for person's own power and self-healing processes
Effective communication	Elements of effective communication	Listen Impart information Learn Facilitate the learning of others Promote and accept patient's emotions	Importance of being open and nonjudgmental

forth. Practitioners must be sensitive to the various communities and develop a sense of working to bring together the best of these communities as they interact with the client/patient and the family. The harmful elements that block a person's healing must be identified and improved to enhance their health and well-being.

The knowledge, skills, and values needed by practitioners to effectively participate in and work with various communities falls

TABLE 1-2 *Health Professions Education and Relationship-Centered Care Patient-Practitioner Relationship: Areas of Knowledge, Skills and Values. Courtesy of PEW Health Professions Commission at the Center for the Health Professions, University of California, San Francisco, California.*

AREA	KNOWLEDGE	SKILLS	VALUES
Meaning of community	Various models of community Myths and misperceptions about community Perspectives from the social sciences, humanities, and systems theory Dynamic change—demographic, political, industrial	Learn continuously Participate actively in community development and dialogue	Respect for the integrity of the community Respect for cultural diversity
Multiple contributors to health within the community	History of community, land use, migration, occupations, and their effect on health Physical, social, and occupational environments and their effects on health External and internal forces influencing community health	Critically assess the relationship of health care providers to community health Assess community and environmental health Assess implications of community policy affecting health	Affirmation of relevance of all determinants of health Affirmation of the value of health policy in community services Recognition of the presence of values that are destructive to health
Developing and maintaining community relationships	History of practitioner-community relationships Isolation of the health care community from the community at large	Communicate ideas Listen openly Empower others Learn Facilitate the learning of others Participate appropriately in community development and activism	Importance of being open-minded Honestly regarding the limits of health science Responsibility to contribute health expertise
Effective community-based care	Various types of care, both formal and informal Effects of institutional scale on care Positive effects of continuity of care	Collaborate with other individuals and organizations Work as member of a team or healing community Implement change strategies	Respect for community leadership Commitment to work for change

into four areas and are summarized in Table 1-2: the meaning of the community; the multiple contributors to health and illness with the community; developing and maintaining relationships with the community; and effective community-based care (Tresolini, 1994).

Practitioner-Practitioner Relationship

In order for nurse healers to provide holistic care for the clients/ patients, families, and significant others, many diverse practitioner-practitioner relationships are involved. To form a practitioner-practitioner relationship requires knowledge, skills, and values related to four areas as summarized in Table 1-3: to develop self-knowledge; to understand traditional knowledge about the diverse knowledge base and skills of different practitioners; to develop team and community building; and to understand the working dynamics of groups, teams, and organizations that can provide resource services for the client/patient, the family, and significant others (Tresolini, 1994). When a true practitioner-practitioner partnership exists, we are vision partners. The qualities of creating vision partnerships are discribed in Figure 1-3, page 11, (Miccoli, 1993).

Practitioners should be aware of the diversity of healing modalities and the different types of practitioners as well as the range of healing modalities that they use. Practitioners must be willing to integrate alternative/complementary practitioners and therapies in the traditional clinic and hospital setting (i.e., relaxation, imagery, music and touch therapies, folk healers, herbs, etc.). This involves continuously learning about the experiences of different healers, different modalities, and valuing cultural diversity.

Strategies for Creating Relationship-Centered Care

Nurse healers are becoming more engaged in the educational and clinical strategies to assist students, practitioners, and educators to evolve relationship-centered care. These strategies must be approached not as competencies or skills to be learned, but more as a new way of being, seeing, and experiencing the healing capacities within oneself. Four strategies are crucial to the process. These are 1) mentorship; 2) non-competitive formative assessments of individuals' educational attainments; 3) support for practitioner

---

TABLE 1-3 *Health Professions Education and Relationship-Centered Care
Patient-Practitioner Relationship: Areas of Knowledge, Skills and Values.
Courtesy of PEW Health Professions Commission at the Center for the Health
Professions, University of California, San Francisco, California.*

AREA	KNOWLEDGE	SKILLS	VALUES
Self-awareness	Knowledge of self	Reflect on self and needs Learn continuously	Importance of self-awareness
Traditions of knowledge in health professions	Healing approaches of various professions Healing approaches across cultures Historical power inequities across professions	Derive meaning from others' work Learn from experience within healing community	Affirmation and value of diversity
Building teams and communities	Perspectives on team-building from the social sciences	Communicate effectively Listen openly Learn cooperatively	Affirmation of mission Affirmation of diversity
Working dynamics of teams, groups, and organizations	Perspectives on team dynamics from the social sciences	Share responsibility responsibly Collaborate with others Work cooperatively Resolve conflicts	Openness to others' ideas Humility Mutual trust, empathy, support Capacity for grace

and educator development; and 4) use of information management and dissemination systems (Tresolini, 1994).

Mentorship. The first learning strategy, mentorship, is at the core
of the learning experience. As nurse healers mentor others they
must share and explore the scientific principles as well as the intuitive hunches that guide practice and the coordination of care.
When this is done then, their philosophy and caring-healing behaviors and attitudes can be modeled. As nurse healers share and
use guided reflections in the mentoring process, those being mentored will experience enhanced self-awareness, values, skills, and
open communication about new possibilities.

Evaluation. The second learning strategy, non-competitive assessments of individuals' education attainment or work performance,

FIGURE 1-3 *Effective Partnering*

VALUES DRIVEN—Partners are driven by values, not by environment, emotions, or circumstances. Do you "walk the talk" of the values you share with your partners?

INTERDEPENDENCE—Interdependence involves the "we" of a partnership. We can do it. We can get there. We can create something greater together. Do you partner with a "we" or a "me" focus?

SHIFTING PARADIGMS—"You can't change the fruit without changing the root." Our paradigms—the models or context in which we do our thinking—frame our attitudes and behaviors. Do you think from the inside out - starting with yourself and putting ethics ahead of personality and popularity? If not, you may need to change your thinking (shift your paradigm). If the fruit is our partnership and the root is how we think, some shifting may be necessary to genuinely achieve your partnership's goals. Are you "root bound"? Do you need to replant your ideas so you can grow better fruit?

INTEGRITY—Integrity is the value we place on ourselves. Personal integrity generates trust by keeping us from judging another before checking our perceptions with that person. Integrity stops us from talking behind another's back; from dishonest communication and behaviors; and from self-serving motivation. Are you honest in your communications? Do you participate in conversations about another person without bringing your concerns to that person directly? Do you voice your convictions even if they are unpopular?

ORGANIZATIONAL OUTCOMES—Focusing on organizational outcomes is a characteristic of organizational excellence. This holds true for partners, too. When partners focus on outcomes, they gain a shared purpose and direction for progress. Are you focused on outcomes and driven by the ones you share with your partner?

NEGOTIATION—In negotiating, partners focus on interests, not positions. A win-win situation is where one partner doesn't succeed at the other's expense. How are your negotiation skills?

PRINCIPLE-CENTERED LEADERSHIP—Principles drive every word, action, and priority of effective partners. Are you a principle-centered leader? Do your actions with your partners reflect your values and principles?

ACCOUNTABILITY—Each of us is accountable to our own effectiveness, for our own happiness, and for most of our circumstances. Are you accountable for your behaviors, words, and priorities in your partnerships?

RENEWAL—With renewal, we can replace old patterns of self-defeating and noncollaborative behavior with new patterns of effectiveness, happiness, and trust. What was the most recent thing you did to renew yourself and your partnerships?

TRUST—Trust nurtures the self-esteem of each partner, enabling him or her to focus on issues rather than personalities and positions. Are you a trust-worthy partner? Do you operate above the table at all times?

NOVELTY—Partnerships are only as much fun and as invigorating as the partners make them. What novel approaches do you use to energize your partnerships?

EVOLUTION—Evolution happens as partners open up the gates for change. Sometimes this may feel like *revolution*, but it's really a gradual metamorphosis toward interdependence in the partnership. Where are your partnerships now compared to where they began?

RESPECT—Only in an environment of mutual respect, where each viewpoint is truly heard, will partners express their most important and truthful thoughts. Are you respectful in your interactions, even in the face of debate and disagreement? Do you listen well without interruption, seeking first to understand before being understood?

SYNERGY—Synergy happens when the combined actions of people working together create a greater effect than each person can achieve alone. Synergistic partnerships value differences, respect them and build on strengths to compensate for weakness. Do your partnerships focus on the contributions of each partner with the goal of creating a greater good for all?

Source: Reprinted from Miccolo, M., Effective Partnering, AACN News, October 1993, with permission of American Association of Colleges of Nursing, © 1993

is an empowering evaluation process that reinforces relationship building between faculty, clinicians, and students. Numerous methods of quantitative and qualitative approaches can be used to assess the depth of attitudes, knowledge, and skills.

Educational Support. The third learning strategy, the ongoing educational strategy of support for practitioners and faculty development, is essential to the learning and development of the skills to be integrated into the healing process. When this strategy is used there is more creativity and the ability of students, practitioners, and faculty to be in an evolving process of healing relationships where one or more individuals are able to be within the mystery of the healing process that has its own time frame (Dossey, et al., 1995; Dossey, et al., 1996).

Information Management. The fourth strategy, the routine use of information management and dissemination systems to inform quality improvement activities to all involved, is important. This incorporates computer-based learning programs, support groups, audiovisual self-paced programs, role playing, sharing stories, and cultural diversity (Flynn, 1995; Goldsmith & Barnsteiner, 1994). This assists clients/patients, practitioners, and faculty in data related to the many factors that influence health-wellness-disease-illness. This includes patterns of practice, established outcomes, the origins of care, and the need for quality improvement activities for patient, communities, and practitioners. Relationship-centered care has important implications for our views of health-wellness-disease-illness because currently technology and the allopathic focus on curing remains very strong. To more fully comprehend another person's story, nurse healers strive to understand the personal meaning inherent in the story.

PERSONAL MEANINGS IN LIVED EXPERIENCES

Nurse healers understand the dynamics of natural systems theory. This theory shows that human beings are living, self-organizing systems that strive for dynamic equilibrium by a continuous information flow within, between others, and the environment (von

Bertalanffy, 1972). From this process personal meanings are derived because individuals have self-organizing abilities that involve mind-modulation, growth, regeneration, learning, healing, and self-transcendence. This mind-modulation, or circular flow of information, allows for sensory information on the state of the individual and the relationship to self, others, and the environment. The field of psychoneuroimmunology has demonstrated that this information flow throughout the body is transmitted via neural networks and receptors in the autonomic, endocrine, immune, and neuropeptide systems to help individuals interpret the meaning of the events experienced (Dossey, 1995).

Nurse healers are challenged to identify the meaning in the clients/patients', families', colleagues' journeys, as well as their own personal journey and those events that inhibit or strengthen healing. All must be active participants in the process. We do not only observe a client/patient, family, or colleague being anxious, afraid, or joyful. The simple act of observation means that we have participated in and perceived signals about the event that impact each of us. This evolving state of expanding consciousness is the process of creating healthier and dynamic patterns in new ways to work and live (Newman, 1995).

Nurse healers recognize that the meanings that a person attaches to symptoms or illness are probably the most important factor influencing the journey of one's life through a crisis. Human beings can view illness from at least eight frames of reference: 1) illness as challenge, 2) illness as enemy, 3) illness as punishment, 4) illness as weakness, 5) illness as relief, 6) illness as strategy, 7) illness as irreparable loss or damage, and 8) illness as value (Lipowski, 1970).

Meanings are individual and personal and they must have congruence with the person's experience, belief systems, rationality, expectations, and the context of the event. Context assumes significance in uncovering meaning and involves a person's past and present life story as well as what one believes about future events (Bevis, 1990). Interpretation and meaning are part of the syntactical category of learning. In syntax one looks at wholes, broad relationships, insights, and patterns and finds or seeks out the meanings. Only when some meaning is found can an experience become a paradigm experience. Meaningless experiences are seldom retained to form a foundation for future reference.

Nurse healers are aware of the importance of recognizing the perception of another as well as their own perception. Perception is an active process and never passive. There are no neutral events and nurse healers are always aware of these interrelated events. For example, an anxious patient is scheduled for an angioplasty within the hour and tells his story about fearing the angioplasty. With focused intention, the nurse healer knows the potential that a person has right in the moment to learn a bodymind intervention that can assist with decreasing the anxiety.

With caring touch the nurse can reach out and hold the patient's hand for a period of time and also take 5 to 10 minutes to teach the patient a relaxing, abdominal breathing exercise. An imagery rehearsal of creating a special place in thoughts and images may also be taught to further help the patient decrease the fear and to cope better with the procedure. The patient might also be given a choice of listening to a relaxation and imagery tape during the procedure. The patient may be offered several different choices of music or a tape that uses relaxation and imagery suggestions that has been specifically created for patients undergoing angioplasty. Following the procedure the patient most often will report decreased anxiety during the procedure and the use of relaxed breathing and imaging a special quiet place as suggested. This patient-nurse healer interaction demonstrates nurse healing and patient-practitioner relationship-centered care. These interventions not only teach the patient skills, but demonstrate the placebo effect that is part of the symbolic and perceived meaning of a therapeutic relationship.

Nurse healers continually reflect on the power of these ordinary interactions in the healing process. They also reflect on the phenomenal question "What does it mean to be human?" (Munhall, 1994). What is meaning? Why should I seek out meaning? What do I do with it? How do I keep it? What does meaning have to do with how I practice? What is the client's/patient's, family's, or significant others' perceived meaning about events?

Meaning is seen as differences, contrasts, novelty, and heterogeneity and is necessary for the healthy function of human beings. Nurse healers seek out meaning because their lives are fuller and richer when they mean something positive. Take away the important meaning of their lives and often it is not worth living. The more individuals understand about meaning in life, the better they are able to empower themselves to recognize effective ways to cope with life and to learn increasingly effective methods of working on life issues. In doing this, nurse healers create richer meaning in their daily lives. This attention to meaning allows them to be more effective with others as they guide them in exploring their personal meanings in daily living.

Nurse healers are aware of the process by which they help clients/patients maintain their sense of meaning and ability to function in the midst of the dynamic changes that may occur with a crisis, in relationships, and within the environment. Being an individual who is faced with a crisis, a critical illness, or a family with a critically ill loved one is to understand the lived experience of this process. It is not the organ system or pathophysiologic condition that has gone awry. For the client/patient, the family, and significant others, health and illness must be viewed as a complex interconnected process.

Nurse healers know that when meaning is absent, human bodies become bored; bored bodies become the spawning ground for depression, disease, and death. Failure of meaning has become a cliché. Professions, personal lives, even entire cultures are said to suffer from a breakdown of meaning. Although at times it seems that meaning may be absent from our lives and our universe, in fact such a thing is not possible, even in principle. What happens is that the meaning has been expressed, suppressed, or forgotten.

Nurse healers are profoundly aware that our existence is awash with meaning and it is only a matter of which meaning each individual shall choose. It is the choices that are crucial. Nowhere is this more important or apparent than in health and illness. It is clear from the wealth of scientific data that it is impossible to separate the biologic parts from the psychologic, sociologic, and spiritual part of our being. The importance of meaning can no longer be ignored for it is directly linked with mind modulation of all body systems that influence states of wellness or illness. Because meanings and emotions go hand in hand, is it strange that the meanings we perceive could affect the body? Or that the body could affect our emotions and our meanings? These connections are so intimate that we must think of the body-mind-spirit as a single integrated unit (Dossey, 1991). A primary assertion for nurse healers as they integrate a holistic model is that consciousness is real and is related to all matters of health-well-ness-disease-illness.

CONCEPTS OF HEALTH-WELLNESS-DISEASE-ILLNESS

To better understand these relationships, it is important to explore the definitions of each (Jensen & Allen, 1993). Health has been defined in many ways such as an ideal state, an integrated balance, and a method of functioning that is oriented toward maximizing the potential of the individual. Wellness has been described as a measure of optimal health, an expression of the process of life, and the subjective experience of integrated or congruent functioning. Disease has varied definitions such as the biological dimensions of non-health or breakdown.

The two prevalent views of disease are that there is an ontological view and a physiologic view (Benner & Wrubel, 1989). In the ontologic view, diseases are seen as some kind of entity in their own right, not as a disturbance or manifestation. In the physiologic view disease is grounded in the nature of human beings, with disease occurring as the result of deviations from the norm or imbalances. Illness is not the absence of health, nor identical to disease. It involves the human experience of symptoms and suffering or the state of being-in-the-world. Illness includes the perceived meaning for the person and how he or she lives within the limitations of the symptoms or of the disability. Thus health-disease and wellness-illness are considered both relational and contextual. Health, disease, wellness, and illness are part of the whole, yet distinct.

Nurse healers are aware of the unfolding of events associated with wellness-illness as a generic paradigm with health, disease, wellness, and illness existing in a dialectic relationship (Jensen & Allen, 1993). This dialectic relationship symbolizes the synthesis of the objective and the subjective perspectives. For example, a person experiencing an angioplasty is not the heart-disease patient, but is a person with an illness related to cardiovascular disease. Following the angioplasty, this person must seriously evaluate and reflect on the life style and events that contributed to this cardiovascular event. The reflective process can assist the patient and the family to decide how to reorganize the patient's life and the family structure in regard to integrating life style changes that can prevent, stabilize, or reverse coronary artery disease (Ornish, 1990).

As nurse healers integrate the art and science of nursing, they are aware that health-disease and wellness-illness are neither mutually exclusive, nor polar opposites, but are part of a process and part of the whole. When an individual is viewed in this way, it is easier to understand that the individual is a changing person in a changing world. Nurse healers are aware of the relationship between health-wellness-disease-illness and the importance of integrating traditional medicine with alternative/complementary therapies.

INTEGRATING ALTERNATIVE/COMPLEMENTARY THERAPIES

Nurse healers are well poised to be active in the integration of many alternative/complementary therapies. These therapies are still not broadly accepted by allopathic medicine. Nurse healers are engaged in clinical practice and research to demonstrate that these modalities work and are cost-effective. Nurse healers recognize the limitations of their nurse practice acts. They also are involved in an ongoing process of providing education to their state nursing boards to have their nurse practice acts revised to reflect holistic nursing practice. Nurse healers are becoming more politically active and provide information and education to policy makers about the cost-effectiveness and enhanced healing with these therapies.

In 1992 the National Institutes of Health (NIH) created the Office of Alternative Medicine (OAM) to evaluate complementary and alternative therapies that capitalize dramatically on mind/body events and healing between individuals and healing at a distance; to identify the therapies that hold the most promise for Americans; and to fund studies evaluating the effectiveness of complementary and alternative therapies. In 1996 the OAM was changed to the Office of Complementary and Alternative Medicine (OCAM) to more accurately reflect their work. The OCAM research budget for 1997 is $11 million.

The purpose of the OCAM is to encourage the investigation of complementary/alternative medical practices, with the ultimate goal of integrating validated complementary and alternative medical practices with current conventional medical practices. Nurse healers have the opportunity to play a major role in the future direction and investigation of many of these complementary and alternative interventions. As more nurse healers integrate the mind/body therapies discussed next, there is more use of the term caring-healing to refer to these interventions.

These complementary and alternative therapies fall into seven fields of practice as described in the Alternative Medicine NIH Report, 1994:

1. mind/body or biobehavioral interventions (biofeedback, relaxation, imagery, meditation, hypnosis, psychotherapy, prayer, art, dance, music therapy, yoga)

2. bioelectromagnetics (BEM) application in medicine (study of various BEM devices and eight new applications of nonthermal, nonionizing EM fields for bone repairs, nerve stimulation, wound healing, osteoarthritis, electroacupuncture, immune system stimulation, neuroendocrine modulation)

3. alternative systems of healing (traditional oriental medicine, acupuncture, ayurvedic medicine, homeopathic medicine, anthroposophically extended medicine, naturopathic medicine, environmental medicine, community-based health care practice [shamans, Native American Indian, AA programs])

4. manual healing methods (osteopathy, massage, cranial-sacral, chiropractic, physical therapy, biofield therapeutics [therapeutic touch, healing touch, Huna, Qigong, Mar-iel, Reiki, kinesiology, polarity])

5. pharmacological and biologic treatments (antineoplastons, cartilage products, EDTA Chelation Therapy, ozone, immunoaugmentative therapy, 714-X, Hoxsey methods, Essiac, Coley's toxins, MTH-68, neural therapy, apitherapy, mistletoe)

6. herbal medicine (various herbs from Europe, China, Asia, India, and Native American Herbal Medicine)

7. diet and nutrition in the prevention of chronic disease (study of various food groups, vitamins, minerals on acute and chronic disease)

It is essential that nurses understand the nurse practice act in their state, however. Because each state nurse practice act is different, the permitted practice of alternative/complementary therapies may vary.

One reason the OCAM was created is that the Federal Government recognized that Americans were pursuing alternative methods of health care with unprecedented enthusiasm. David M. Eisenberg, M.D., of Harvard Medical School and Beth Israel Hospital, and his colleagues described this current trend in an article, "Unconventional Medicine in the United States," published in *The New England Journal of Medicine.* They found that in 1990 about one third of all American adults sought out alternative medicine of some variety (Eisenberg, 1993). This involved 425 million visits to practitioners of alternative medicine, which exceeded the total number of visits to primary care physicians in the United States. Expenditures for alternative care were $14 billion, most of which was out-of-pocket, and unreimbursed by insurance plans.

One of the most interesting findings of Eisenberg's study was that over 70 percent of persons seeking alternative/complementary therapies care chose not to inform their allopathic physicians. This may help explain why many allopathic physicians believe the fuss over alternative measures is a tempest in a teapot; they simply are unaware of what their patients are doing. Skeptics frequently charge that persons interested in alternative/complementary medicine are economically deprived and poorly educated, thus easily misled. The Eisenberg study found the opposite in that alternative/complementary consumers tend to be educated, upper-income whites in the 25 to 49 age group.

Nurse healers advocate a "both/and" instead of an "either/or" approach in interfacing complementary alternative therapies with traditional medical and surgical therapies. Complementary/alternative therapies must be considered as adjuncts or complements to conventional biotechnology and pharmacology and not as a replacement for them. However, many health care practitioners and laypersons are asking if healing can take place in our hospitals, clinics, rehabilitation centers, and home health care while most parts of the current health care system continue to be a disease management industry.

As nurse healers expand their role in addressing the body-mind-spirit dimensions of individuals, they serve as models of how healing can enter into the health care arena. They are exploring the scientific data and acquiring the knowledge and skills to integrate both the art and science of holistic nursing practice. Nurse healers are at the forefront of the dramatic and dynamic changes that are occurring in health care delivery.

REFERENCES

Alternative Medicine: Expanding Medical Horizons. (Chantilly, VA: NIH Report No. 94-066, 1994.

American Holistic Nurses' Association. (1994a). *Working description of holistic nursing.* Raleigh, NC.

American Holistic Nurses' Association. (1997b). *Standards of holistic nursing practice.* Raleigh, NC.

Benner, P., & Wrubel, J. (1989). *The primacy of caring.* Menlo Park, CA: Addison-Wesley Publishing Company.

Bevis, E. O. (1990). Accessing learning: Determining worth or developing excellence—from a behaviorist toward an interpretative-criticism model. In E. O. Bevis and J. Watson (Ed.), *Toward a caring curriculum: A new pedagogy for nursing.* New York: National League for Nursing Press.

Dossey, B., Keegan, L., Guzzetta, C., & Kolkmeier, L. (1995). *Holistic nursing: A handbook for practice* (2nd ed.). Gaithersburg, MD: Aspen Publishers, Inc.

Dossey, B., Keegan, L., & Guzzetta, C. (1996). *The art of caring: Using relaxation, imagery, music therapy, and touch.* Boulder, CO: Sounds True.

Dossey, L. (1991). *Meaning and medicine.* New York: Bantam Books.

Eisenberg, D.M., Kessler, R. C., Foster, C., Norlock, F. E., Calkins, D., & Delbanco, T. L. (1993, January 28). Unconventional medicine in the United States. *New England Journal of Medicine, 328* (4), 246–252.

Flynn, J. (1995). Shifting paradigms. *Nursing Leadership Forum, 1* (1).

Goldsmith, J., & Barnsteiner, J. (1994). Pyramiding knowledge into practice. *Reflections, 6.*

Jensen, L., & Allen, M. (1993). *Wellness: The dialect of illness. Image, 25* (3), 220–224.

Keegan, L. (1994). *Nurse as healer.* Albany, NY: Delmar Publishers Inc.

Lipowski, Z. J. (1970). Physical illness, the individual and the coping process. *Psychiatric Medicine,* 1, 90.

Miccoli, M. (1993). *Effective partnering.* Aliso Viejo, CA: AACN News, p. 2.

Munhall, P. (1994). *Revisioning phenomenology: Nursing and health science research.* New York: National League for Nursing Press.

Newman, M. (1995). *Health as expanding consciousness.* New York: The National League for Nursing Press.

OAM Report. (1995). *Alternative Therapies in Health and Medicine, 1* (2), 16.

Ornish, D. (1990). Can lifestyle reverse coronary heart disease? *Lancet,* 336, 129–46.

Tresolini, C. P., & the Pew-Fetzer Task Force. (1994). *Health professions education and relationship-centered care.* San Francisco, CA: Pew Health Professions Commission.

von Bertalanffy, L. (1972). *General systems theory.* New York: George Braziller, Inc.

THE EVOLUTION OF NURSE HEALERS

2 | THE EVOLUTION OF NURSE HEALERS

INTRODUCTION

As we stand at the doorstep of the twenty-first century, nurse healers are creating and integrating new caring-healing models that guide in the healing of self and others (Watson, 1988; Benner & Wrubel, 1985). Caring is a human mode of being that is a basic element of being a person. When we do not care, we seem to lose our "being." However, the "Five C's of Caring" can help us in our caring-healing practices and life (Mayeroff, 1972). These are compassion, competence, confidence, conscience, and commitment.

THE CARING-HEALING PROCESS

Compassion is a way of being that can be enhanced as we develop our inner awareness of our various relationships with self and others. This also involves our connections with all living things such as plants, animals, and all aspects of the living and nonliving world.

Competence is that state of recognizing and gaining knowledge, judgment, skills, energy, experience, and motivation. These aspects are required in order for us to respond adequately to the demands of our professional responsibilities.

Confidence is the quality that fosters the building of trusting relationships. It requires attention and time alone to reflect on many aspects of being human. Confidence comes with experience and taking risks and enables us to change our world view when the old ways no longer serve us.

Conscience is a state of moral awareness. It is when we adhere to a professional ethic of caring and healing that seeks to improve the dignity and wholeness of the person and the family who is receiving care. This also implies our own personal ethic in how we live our lives.

Commitment is a complex and affective response. It is characterized by a convergence of one's values, desires, and obligations and by a deliberate choice to act in accordance with them.

Eight additional qualities have also been identified within caring (Roach, 1987). These are knowledge, alternating rhythms, patience, honesty, trust, humility, hope, and courage.

Knowledge about another person is essential if we are to identify the person's needs and what interventions will help in healing. It is also necessary for us to know our own strengths and limitations. We must recognize cognitive knowledge as well as intuitive knowledge, because both are important aspects of the caring-healing process.

Alternative rhythms refers to the past, present, and future situations that we move between and among. It involves the narrow and the wide frameworks between attention to details and attention to the whole. Both of these are necessary and both are part of caring.

Patience involves who we are in the moment, of not doing, but being with what may evolve. This does not mean that we wait passively for something to happen. It means giving attention while allowing the person to go at their own pace in the decision-making and the learning process.

Honesty is how we learn to tell the truth to ourselves in various situations. This is a positive, often active event where we try to bring consensus to a situation and to release confrontation. We use our skills of active listening so that we can understand another person's perception and not what we would like the person to do.

Trusting allows us to come from a place in our caring-healing interactions where we are there to assist another. This involves the appreciation of the other person. Often we can get caught in trying to care too much and overprotect others, thus we lose sight of a co-participating relationship in the decision and evaluation processes.

Humility helps us with how we see others as existing for themselves, not simply to satisfy our needs. When we treat each person and each situation as unique, we relate with humility to each event.

Hope is a process of caring that is always present. Yet in a crisis or during illness, it may be forgotten. Hope is not wishful thinking, but it is an expression of the fullness of presence that allows the unfolding for healing outcomes.

Courage is the capacity to go into the unknown. It allows us and others to take risks about different choices. Courage is not blind. It is informed by knowledge and intuition about past, present, and future possibilities. It helps us build trust in our own inner wisdom and to build trust in the ability of others to change and grow. As these concepts are interwoven in the caring-healing process, we are more present to truly be nurse healers.

NURSE AS HEALER

A nurse who is healing is a nurse who helps facilitate another's growth toward wholeness—body-mind-spirit—or who assists with recovery from illness or with transition to peaceful death. Reflect for a moment on the characteristics of a nurse that facilitates healing in self, patients, and others (Dossey, 1995c):

- Awareness that self-healing is a continual process
- Familiarity with the terrain of self-development
- Recognition of weaknesses and strengths
- Openness to self-discovery
- Continued effort to develop clarity about life's purposes to avoid mechanical behavior and boredom
- Awareness of present and future steps in personal growth
- Modeling of self-care in order to help self and clients with the process of inner reflection of life's meanings and priorities
- Awareness that a nurse's presence is as important as technical skills

- Respect and love for patients regardless of who or how they are

- Willingness to offer the patient methods for working on life issues

- Ability to guide the client in discovering creative options

- Presumption that the client knows the best life choices

- Active listening

- Empowerment of client to recognize that they can cope with life processes

- Sharing of insights without imposing personal values and beliefs

- Acceptance of what clients say without judging

- Perception of time with clients as being there to serve and share with them

Developing the characteristics of a nurse healer moves us in the direction of life's purpose. Purpose implies a conscious direction toward maximizing human potential. Increasing purpose in one's life can be achieved along two dimensions of growth—the personal and the transpersonal (Dossey, 1995c). The personal dimension of growth concerns meaning and integration of our personal existence. This dimension—possessing logical and analytical thought and being self-motivated and goal-oriented in one's professional and personal life—is what is most valued in Western culture. The transpersonal dimension is less recognized and valued in Western culture, however, it is just as important. This dimension concerns the ultimate meaning and purpose of the universal existence of humanity. We should also consider a third dimension of human growth, the interpersonal dimension, which is part of the other two dimensions. In the personal dimension one develops the basic social skills of communication, courtesy, and friendship that are requisite for survival with others. As we begin to develop along the transpersonal dimension, we become aware of our basic interdependency, the essential merging with the other. The merging of the interpersonal with the other two dimensions allows us to have balanced, supportive relationships with family, friends, community, and patients. It also allows the depth necessary in meaningful relationships. Without the interpersonal dimension, our relationships would be at best unenlightened and superficial.

As nurses integrate their personal, interpersonal, and transpersonal dimensions they have more capacity for responsibility and choice in the moment and in life as a whole. They recognize a sense of having a destiny, a meaning, and an overall purpose in life. There is true preference for living in accordance with one's purpose(s) so that when different distractions or conflicts arise they are more easily recognized. Thus, we are more willing to accept the limitations of one's life and to be in the world just as it is.

HEALING VERSUS CURING

The health care system focus for the last twenty-five years has been on curing of symptoms in a masculine, allopathic model. Curing has been associated with power, analysis of data, and technology, whereas healing has had little status and few financial rewards. Current information necessitates that we mesh curing and healing for the most effective results.

In order to achieve this we must call for a redefinition of healing (Achterberg, Dossey, & Kolkmeier, 1994). Healing is a life-long journey into understanding the wholeness of human existence. Along this journey, our lives blend with those of our clients, their families, and our colleagues where moments of new meaning and insight emerge in the midst of crisis. Healing occurs when we embrace and transform what is feared or most painful in our lives, when we remember what has been forgotten about connection, and unity and interdependence. Healing is learning how to open what has closed so that we can expand our inner human potentials. True healing is entering into the transcendent, timeless moment when one experiences a connection with a divinity or the universe. Healing involves creativity, passion, love, and learning to trust life. It is seeking and expressing self in its fullness, its light and shadow, its masculine and feminine.

A healing system is an interconnected web replete with feminine energy as contrasted to the more common models of linear, hierarchical relationships which is a masculine order of thought (Achterberg, 1990). This healing system has bonds among and within levels which are invisible and nonmaterial. These bonds are the healing forces of the human spirit—love, compassion, motivation, conscious and unconscious thought, purpose, and will. Each level of the healing system demands a technology and a data base about the bio-psycho-social-spiritual domains. The challenges are to integrate feminine values with masculine standards; to couple flexibility with decisiveness, perspective with focus, synthesis with analysis.

What will it take for healing and the human spirit to emerge with the current emphasis on technology and curing? Many people are ready to change destructive life-style habits that lead to imbalance and illness. Individuals now recognize that both allopathic approaches and healing modalities are needed to stabilize or reverse disease and to improve their quality of life.

It is time that professionals honor their masculine and feminine voices. As men and women learn to respect the balance of these qualities as listed in Table 2-1, healing will begin to emerge in our health care system.

TABLE 2-1   *Examples of Masculine and Feminine Qualities*

MASCULINE	FEMININE
Intellect	Intuition
Linear	Nonlinear
How	Why
Knowledge	Wisdom
Power	Compassion
Analysis	Synthesis
Expansive	Contained
Proactive	Reactive
Giving	Receiving
External/public	Internal/private
Technical	Natural
Form	Process
Competition	Collaboration
Objective	Subjective
Doing to	Being with
Curing	Caring
Fixing	Nurturing
Reason	Feelings
Physical world	Invisible world
Decisive	Flexible

Source: Adapted from *Woman as Healer* by J. Achterberg, p. 191, with permission of Shambhala Publications, Inc., © 1990.

As nurses, both male and female, understand the importance of the feminine voice, there will emerge a reawakening of spirit in clinical practice. Spirituality is directly related to inner knowing and source of strength reflected in one's being, one's knowing, and one's doing (Burkhardt & Nagai-Jacobson, 1994). We must continue to learn to be in dialogue with each other to remember the wisdom of "doing what we know" and "knowing what we do," and continue to move toward balancing our feminine and masculine qualities. Nurses have been so buried in the layers of patriarchal learning and conditioning that the doing and knowing has been difficult. Nurses must motivate each other and learn to honor and talk about their healing interactions. Within the context of community, when nurses honor each other it is affirming, encouraging, stimulating, and exciting. Nurses are then in a position to share the peace and power about themselves and their healing work.

Healing and caring have emerged as the essence of nursing and the central, dominant, and unifying feature of nursing. From one comparative analysis of conceptualizations and theories of caring five major themes have been identified: caring as a human trait, caring as a moral imperative, caring as an affect interaction, caring as an interpersonal interaction, and caring as a therapeutic intervention (Morse, 1991). Outcomes of caring are categorized as the patient's subjective experience, the patient's physical response, and the nurse's subjective experience.

Presently, the concepts of healing and caring need more scientific investigation, clarity of definitions, and a healthy debate in nursing. The levels of knowledge, theory, and research needed in a practice-oriented discipline must be considered in relation to different aspects of reality. As we expand our models we create new paradigms that recognize a spectrum of reality from "body" through "mind" to "spirit," which provided more of a philosophical basis for understanding the necessity of multiple modes of inquiry and multiple types of knowledge and theory. With this type of thinking we are in a position to see and experience the complementary rather than the competitive, the inherently superior, or the inferior (Wolfer, 1993).

This healing system calls for recognition by the professional of the aspects of being a "wounded healer." This implies that each professional must acknowledge the inner work that must occur in one's spiritual dimension. Our wounds, and the wounds of the medical system, are very similar in that the reintegration of the feminine principle, the feminine perspective, is a major step in our own personal healing and the healing of the medical system (Remen, 1993). We must focus not on curing, but on healing and the laws of healing. This creates personal transformation where the professional is more available to help others through crisis, transition, and to facilitate the healing process. Recognizing our wounded healer sets us on a healing path that moves us in understanding the evolving process towards wholeness and healing. The continual process of healing ourselves is the first step in facilitating healing in others. As nurse healers continue to increase their own awareness of how their bodies and minds interact they more quickly recognize the mind-body dilemma that is present in allopathic medicine as discussed next.

ADDRESSING THE MIND-BODY DILEMMA

Nurse healers are aware of the focus in traditional settings about how the mind is separated from the body with most allopathic therapies. The relationship between mind and body has been called one of the most difficult philosophical problems in the history of Western medicine. Until recently it was fashionable to embrace the reductionistic view and reject any approach centering on the relationship between mind and body. However, increasingly potent forms of physical, psychological, social, and spiritual interventions have surfaced outside of mainstream medicine that can no longer be ignored by Western medicine.

Allopathic approaches focus on the anatomic, physiologic, cellular, molecular, genetic, and pharmacological scientific methods of decreasing, stabilizing, or reversing disease. This focus has concentrated solely on the body side of the body-mind equation. Data are now available to assist health care professionals to understand the way the mind and body are connected and how they communicate (Dossey, 1995a). We now know that complementary and alternative therapies also can be used to help individuals to access their inner healing resources. This knowledge may provide the missing link in treating patients. After all these centuries, the body approach to treating illness may have missed the mark because it has not taken into account the profound, devastating effects nor the enormous healing effects of the mind. Treating body ailments with body-oriented therapies may be only half of the answer. There is an increase in significant outcomes when both sides of the body-mind-spirit equation are addressed.

The role of nurse healers is clear. We need to learn to incorporate complementary and alternative therapies to treat physiologic as well as the psychological and spiritual sequelae inherent to all illness. In addition, however, we need to learn to supplement the best of traditional medical therapies with the best of mind therapies as a means of activating inner healing, thus augmenting the effects of drugs, surgery, and technologic therapies. The results could revolutionize the way care is delivered and may significantly improve morbidity and mortality rates and the quality of life. When these changes are integrated, the essence of real healing will be unveiled.

Addressing the Human Spirit in Healing

Nurse healers are aware that spiritual well-being is at the core of meaning and healing. When we address spiritual well-being we assist patients in accessing their inner healing resources of hope, strength, faith, connections, etc. Three areas that are integral to the spiritual well-being of clients are care practitioners, family/friends, and religion/faith (Clark & Heidenreich, 1995). Nursing interventions identified for the three areas include establishing trusting relationships, providing in-depth spiritual assessment, conveying technical competence, and acting as facilitator among family, clergy, and other practitioners. Due to variations in health status and environmental factors, clients' perceptions of hope and well-meaning may change. Therefore, nurses should conduct spiritual assessment, both on admission and intermittently throughout the hospital stay, during clinic visits, home health care visits, and in private practice settings.

Burkhardt synthesized 109 nursing articles and research studies on the concept of spirit and spirituality (Burkhardt, 1989). From her synthesis, she found that spirit and spirituality are frequently linked to religiosity. Thus, the use of the participle, spiriting, is more representative of the concept of spirit. Her synthesis reveals that this spiriting concept falls into four main categories: spirit/spirituality, spiritual dimension, spiritual well-being, and spiritual needs.

From these categories, the following three defining characteristics of spirituality evolved: unfolding mystery, inner strengths, and harmonious interconnectedness. Unfolding mystery refers to one's experience about life's purpose and meaning, mystery, uncertainty, and struggles. Inner strengths refer to a sense of awareness, self, consciousness, inner resources, sacred source, unifying force, inner core, and transcendence. Harmonious interconnectedness includes the connections and relationships, and harmony with self, others, higher power/God, and the environment.

An assessment tool that is organized by the three defining characteristics of spirituality just discussed is seen in Figure 2-1 (Dossey & Guzzetta, 1995). The tool is divided into three categories: meaning and purpose, inner strengths, and interconnections. This tool provides reflective questions for assessing, evaluating, and increasing awareness of spirituality in clients, families, and self. The reflective questions in this tool can facilitate healing because they stimulate spontaneous, independent, meaningful initiatives to improve the individual's capacity for recovery and healing.

Use of bio-psycho-social-spiritual tools and integration of complementary and alternative therapies also assist nurses in meeting the mandate by the Joint Commission on Accreditation of Health care Organizations (JCAHO) to deliver the Patient Bill of Rights and to improve the quality of health care. The Patient Bill of Rights (RI.1.1.2) states that "care of the patient must include consideration of the psychosocial, spiritual, and cultural variables that influence the perception of illness. The provision of patient care reflects consideration of the patient as an individual with personal values and belief systems that impact upon his/her attitude and response to the care that is provided by the organization" (Patient Rights, 1992).

Addressing a Kinder, Gentler Setting for Caring and Healing

Acute, chronic, long term care units, and clinics can be designed in a superb manner to deal with physiologic crisis, constant surveillance, and technologic treatment (Dracup & Bryan-Brown, 1995). However, we also need to view the hospital, clinic, and other settings through the eyes of the patient, family, and significant others.

SPIRITUAL ASSESSMENT TOOL

To facilitate the healing process in clients/patients, families, significant others, and yourself, the following reflective questions assist in assessing, evaluating, and increasing awareness of the spiritual process in yourself and others.

MEANING AND PURPOSE

These questions assess a person's ability to seek meaning and fulfillment in life, manifest hope, and accept ambiguity and uncertainty.

- What gives your life meaning?
- Do you have a sense of purpose in life?
- Does your illness interfere with your life goals?
- Why do you want to get well?
- How hopeful are you about obtaining a better degree of health?
- Do you feel that you have a responsibility in maintaining your health?
- Will you be able to make changes in your life to maintain your health?
- Are you motivated to get well?
- What is the most important or powerful thing in your life?

INNER STRENGTHS

These questions assess a person's ability to manifest joy and recognize strengths, choices, goals and faith.

- What brings you joy and peace in your life?
- What can you do to feel alive and full of spirit?
- What traits do you like about yourself?
- What are your personal strengths?
- What choices are available to you to enhance your healing?
- What life goals have you set for yourself?
- Do you think that stress in any way caused your illness?
- How aware were you of your body before you became sick?
- What do you believe in?
- Is faith important in your life?
- How has your illness influenced your faith?
- Does faith play a role in recognizing your health?

INTERCONNECTIONS

These questions assess a person's positive self-concept, self-esteem, and sense of self; sense of belonging in the world with others; capacity to pursue personal interest; and ability to demonstrate love of self and self-forgiveness.

- How do you feel about yourself right now?
- How do you feel when you have a true sense of you?
- Do you pursue things of personal interest?
- What do you do to show love for yourself?
- Can you forgive yourself?
- What do you do to heal your spirit?

FIGURE 2-1 Spiritual Assessment Tool

These questions assess a person's ability to connect in life-giving ways with family, friends, and social groups and to engage in the forgiveness of others.
- Who are the significant people in your life?
- Do you have friends or family in town who are available to help you?
- Who are the people to whom you are closest?
- Do you belong to any groups?
- Can you ask people for help when you need it?
- Can you share your feelings with others?
- What are some of the most loving things that others have done for you?
- What are the loving things that you do for other people?
- Are you able to forgive others?

These questions assess a person's capacity for finding meaning in worship or religious activities and a connectedness with a divinity or universe.
- Is worship important to you?
- What do you consider the most significant act of worship in your life?
- Do you participate in any religious activities?
- Do you believe in God or a higher power?
- Do you think that prayer is powerful?
- Have you ever tried to empty your mind of all thoughts to see what the experience might be?
- Do you use relaxation or imagery skills?
- Do you meditate?
- Do you pray?
- What is your prayer?
- How are your prayers answered?
- Do you have a sense of belonging in this world?

These questions assess a person's ability to experience a sense of connection with all of life and nature, an awareness of the effects of the environment on life and well-being, and a capacity or concern for the health of the environment.
- Do you ever feel at some level a connection with the world or universe?
- How does your environment have an impact on your state of well-being?
- What are your environment stressors at work and at home?
- Do you incorporate strategies to reduce your environmental stressors?
- Do you have any concerns for the state of your immediate environment?
- Are you involved with environmental issues such as recycling environmental resources at home, work, or in your community?
- Are you concerned about the survival of the planet?

Source: Based on Margaret Burkhardt: Spirituality: An analysis of the concept, *Holistic Nursing Practice* 3(3):69. 1989.

Dossey, B., Keegan, L., Guzzetta, C., and Kolkmeier, L. *Holistic Nursing: A Handbook for Practice*, 2nd ed. (Gaithersburg, MD: Aspen Publishers, 1995).

FIGURE 2-1 Spiritual Assessment Tool (continued)

What barriers exist to physical access? How can we personalize the patient and his or her environment? What are the existing visiting hours if in the hospital? How do we integrate the family and significant others into the patient's care? Are patients being given opportunities to experience relaxation, imagery, music, and touch interventions to decrease pain, anxiety, and fear? Is self-paced learning via audiotapes or video being used for patients in the hospital or on an outpatient basis with clients that are ready to learn about the present or next step in the recovery and healing process? Is pet therapy being used? What kind of healing rituals are being offered to help the patient or client and loved ones to employ and empower their healing resources? Are concerned family members being assessed and given the option of being escorted into a room to see their loved one during a cardiac arrest code for a few minutes if this is their desire? How do we care for patients who will probably not be discharged from the hospital?

Despite biotechnological advances 70% of individuals in the United States still die in institutions, many of them in the critical care unit. As patients seen in hospitals seem to be more critically ill due to changes in length of hospital stay or criteria for being admitted to hospitals, we are faced with striving for clinical excellence with limited time and resources. What do we do when we are faced with the privilege of being with patients in their final moments to help them die with dignity, comfort, and serenity? How do we ensure that patients and their families know about the Self-Determination Act and what is being done to help them make care choices and decisions to forgo life-sustaining treatment? (President's Commision for the Study of Ethical Problems in Medicine and Biomedical and Behavioral Research, 1994) (Harvey, 1994).

How do we help the family and friends, or each other with the discomforts of dying such as sadness and grief? Is the environment of the family room comfortable? Are there support services such as beepers for families who wish to leave the hospital and go out to dinner or home to rest? How often are families and significant others given the names and numbers of support groups to help them through the crisis? How have hospital volunteers been organized to help families in crisis? Crisis and illness creates many levels of uncertainty. Nurse healers understand the need to recognize both the knowing and unknowing inherent within all situations.

Addressing Patterns of Knowing and Unknowing

Nurses are broadening their experience of themselves as healers and becoming vocal about what they need to practice the healing arts in nursing. Carper (1978) identified four knowledge patterns essential to professional nursing. These patterns can empower nurses to recognize their unique qualities. These patterns of knowing—empirical knowledge, personal knowledge, ethical knowledge, and aesthetic knowledge—lead to a form of confidence that is invaluable if new aspects of reality and the true philosophy and science of caring and healing are to emerge. A state of knowing may bring to a halt a further exploration of intuition and unknown areas, however. Munhall (1993) challenges nurses to a new pattern called "unknowing." The state of mind and the "art" of unknowing leads to a state of openness and authenticity where a nurse can admit to self and another, "I don't know you and your subjective world." This coming together of two people that creates a phenomenal field clearly focuses on the intersubjective space where all sources of human understanding, empathy, and conflict can more easily evolve. It is in this state of unknowing that nurse as healer is manifest in the deepest sense. As both nurse and client integrate patterns of knowing and the pattern of unknowing, conceptual frameworks of caring can be demonstrated and not simply proclaimed.

Awareness of one's own spirituality and intentionally caring for one's own spirit are important components in the process of integrating spirituality into personal and professional practice. Knowing as well as unknowing ourselves leads to relating to others, with the outcome being more meaningful relationships. We are more likely to attune to our life purposes and our unique qualities that we bring into our work. As we do this we become more present with ourselves and others.

Addressing Presence

Understanding the concept of presence has significant implications for nurse healers in all areas of practice, education, and research. A common recurring definition and use of the word *presence* is being. Being as a noun is commonly defined as "existence" and "actuality." A synonym for being is essence. Two components of presence have been identified: the physical "being there" and the psychological "being with" that includes the nurse's use of spirituality, individuality, and authenticity (Gilje, 1992).

Presence is the state achieved when one moves within oneself to an inner reference of stability. It is a sense of self-relatedness that can be thought of as a place of inner being, a place of quietude within where one can feel truly integrated, unified, and focused (McKivergin, 1994). Presence is a personal space apart from either involvement or the consequent reaction to that involvement. To be present implies a quality and essence of being in the moment.

Presence means daily integrating solitude to quiet the inner dialogue and body simultaneously and learning to experience sensations in the body-mind-spirit. This can be enhanced through practice of various biobehavioral modalities such as relaxation, imagery, and music or meditative disciplines. One of the most powerful ways to become present with self and others is through the breath. When we are not in the present moment, our breathing is usually high and shallow in the chest, referred to as fight-or-flight breathing, the "I (ego)-self." However when we drop from shallow chest breathing down to abdominal breathing, one's consciousness changes from I-centered to essence-centered breathing (Hendricks & Hendricks, 1993). This essence-centered breathing can bring us into a state of presence. It is as if a loop of awareness occurs where new insight and healing can evolve and can be created in any interaction. This happens because intention flows more easily between nurse and client.

When we develop the skills and awareness of presence, our ability to become more sensitive to our life patterns and processes increases. We act more frequently with purposeful intention. We have a greater ability to be with our state of resolution; that is, we are more willing to experience and face our fears and worries. Presence allows us to devote more time to be silent within. This quality of inner silence lets us understand more about our inner wisdom. A place of presence helps us gain access to when we acknowledge our polarities in life. Our love flows naturally, for we are open to the expressions of nonjudgmental love when we expand our consciousness (Newman, 1994). When this quality is integrated in our lives we are more consistently available for meaningful relationships.

Presence helps us achieve a state of basic vulnerability. This basic vulnerability is a space where we release the outer shell or facade of our roles. Ordinarily we identify the self we know from an awareness of our different roles and our constant stream of thoughts and feelings. Within this space of inner quietude we learn to fall into the space between the successive moments of trying to grasp onto ideas and feelings. It is in this space that we open to being with others in a different way.

Presence allows us to enter into a place of conflict. As we learn the importance of this work we can assist clients, families, and colleagues to also acknowledge the place of conflict. We are able to see the polarity that resides in conflict. The most effective way we can identify conflict is by recognizing its opposite, resolution. We are better able to organize inner energy and balance it with the incoming energy of people and events.

Presence creates the possibility to activate true healing because the nurse is empty of personal needs, especially the need to be a good nurse or to have the right technique or say the right thing. The term *psychotherapeutic jargon* is helpful. This refers to the things that interfere with self-healing. Presence in the moment allows the release of the guilt and frustration of "I don't have time to do the important teaching that I should be doing" or "If only I had time to be with the patient." Learning the skills of how to be more fully present allows the nurse to be able to spend five to ten focused minutes with a client and share ideas that may be a marked turning point in the individual's self-healing. For example, spending a few moments teaching a client breathing and relaxation techniques to decrease anxiety may be the beginning of self-discovery that can lead to awakening his or her healing potential. This period of focused intention with a client may be as valuable as or more valuable than an hour of counseling.

Our basic work as nurse healers is to become full human beings and to inspire full human-beingness in other people. When we are present, we experience wholeness that vibrates and radiates from us. Being present basically means a spirited presence, an intunement with the situation and the capacity to absorb, process, do, or simply be in the unknowing. It involves a spiritual transcendence where one experiences oneself in relationship as a part of a force greater than oneself that is a source of energy for caring. It is learning that narrow path between healthy enmeshment and inappropriate distance on the others (Barnsteiner, Gillis-

Donovan, Knox-Fischer, & McKlindon, 1994). The transcendence of the ego allows nurse healers to become deeply involved without succumbing to destructive forms of overinvolvement.

As we place a prime value on being there with full presence, the clinical environment can change (Karl, 1992). Who do you bring to your practice? What conditions enable you to be there with full presence? What sources sustain, inspire, support, and nourish you to be there well? How can nurses be there well when the caring values of nurses frequently are in opposition to the norms within the traditional clinical setting? In many clinical settings the perception is that nursing is a medically driven, delegated workload. However, a key to transforming this perspective and managing the issue of workload intensity perception may be in delineating the work that needs to be done in caring for patients. As nurses develop consensual standards of care that focus on independent caring aspects of nursing, presence and healing are integrated into realities of clinical practice (Watson, 1988). If a caring-healing practice is to be sustained in all clinical settings, administration must provide opportunities for healthy dialogue and time to develop frameworks and standards, and must mold the organizational cultural context that reflects a paradigm shift of caring-healing models and language (Montgomery, 1992).

Addressing The Art of Guiding

A nurse healer is a guide who uses the art of guiding to help others discover and recognize new health behaviors, make choices, and discover insights about how to cope more effectively (Keegan, 1994). A guide also helps a person explore purpose and meaning in life. Guiding is a special art and a healing intervention that one may use at all times. We must remember that although a person may be critically ill, that individual still possesses inner healing. Within the midst of crisis, patients often forget their innate healing resources and need to be guided and assisted to remember ways that they have gotten through crisis before and what sustains them. Healing is easier to evoke when we give space to enter into a state of intention. This provides more opportunities to be with another to bring to the present moment a person's fullest potential. Being present helps the individual be in congruence with his or her inner resources, to decrease stress, and to enhance self-direction toward balance and harmony. A nurse healer guides the individual in developing all areas of human potential about the inner journey of self-discovery, but the nurse as guide does not assume to know what is the best course for the person. Individuals must make their own choices. As patients and clients seek guidance and help with life possibilities and dilemmas, the nurse as a guide knows some of the hazards and precautions that occur within crisis and trauma, but can only suggest new strategies and options. The nurse has no way of knowing what each experience holds for a person, for moment by moment, the contrast of polarities, such as health and illness, joy and sadness, are always present in one's life.

Addressing Real versus Pseudo-Listening

Good listening is achieved by the ability of the nurse to quiet the person's inner dialogue. Good listening has an enormous quality of nowness. Nowness is the ability to throw away intellectualizations when the client goes off in an unexpected direction. How often, when counseling a client who is intent on telling a part of his or her story, does the nurse stop the flow of the story and bring the person back to a certain point which then may block the client's insight. Often we get too intent on a personal viewpoint of what we think should be happening, because we start our own inner dialogue of analysis and intellectualization. As we increase this process of nowness, it allows the client also to move to a state of nowness that provides a place of inner wisdom to emerge. Questioning and listening that does not structure the answers, except minimally, is a great art.

Any communication process has three components. These are: a sender of the message, a receiver of the message, and the content of the material. In order for us to understand others, we must listen actively (Dossey, 1995c). Being quiet while someone else is talking is not equivalent to real listening. The key to real listening is intention. Intention occurs when we focus with someone in order to move with purpose in our responses and interventions. This can lead others or ourselves toward effective action steps or forward in personal growth. Real listening occurs when we have the intention to understand someone, enjoy someone, learn something, or want to give help to someone.

At times, we all lapse into pseudo-listening when we try to meet the needs of others. Some signs of pseudo-listening that indicate we are meeting personal needs and not listening actively are (Dossey, 1995c):

- silence as you buy time preparing your next remark
- listening to others so that they will listen to you
- listening only to specific information while deleting the rest
- acting interested when you are not
- partially listening because you do not want to disappoint another person
- listening in order not to be rejected
- searching for a person's weaknesses in order to take advantage of them
- identifying weak points in dialogue so that you can be stronger in your response.

We must continue to learn how to be with others. The first focus is to learn to listen actively to what is going on with another person. The second focus is to enable the individual to live in what is, not to avoid it, to let it be. Active listening skills promote effective communication in several ways. The message can be clarified. The receiver of the message can verify nonverbal messages communicated through body language or by what is not said by the sender of the message. The receiver is also able to gather additional information that can help with interventions. Active listening facilitates a greater acceptance of the sender's thoughts and emotions. Thus, the receiver of the message may be in a better situation to choose the most effective behaviors that lead toward health and wholeness.

Addressing Our Relationships with Others

As nurse healers engage in holistic nursing and embark on their inward journey for self-change we must recognize that what we communicate by word, act, attitude, and setting will affect our potential for change (Peper & Kushel, 1985). We must be present oriented and consciously learn the skills to stay in the present moment because change takes place in the present, not in the past or future. Everything affects our clients, our choice of words, our presence, and our greeting. Our beliefs are important and affect our self-image which in turn affects our actions. It also influences our capacity for self-healing.

Our beliefs are conveyed to our clients. We must perceive ourselves and the client as whole. We must remember that the nurse and the client are whole and not a portion of disturbance or pathology. When we perceive the heart patient as a person with heart disease we release the label. We encourage pathology when we focus primarily on it and not on the person's healing potential.

Every part is connected to every other part, and every part in the system affects every other part. We form a network in which everyone participates. There is no such thing as an independent observer. When two people come together they are always creating change in one another.

We must consider the life patterns and situations that the individual is confronting. Look at all the person's life potentials—physical, mental, emotional, spiritual, relationships, and choices. It is only when we consider the whole person and their significant others that we have a chance at facilitating the client toward wholeness. We must continue to gain new skills and become self-experienced in all modalities that we offer to the client. We cannot guide clients down new paths to new experiences if we do not know the path from experience. The more we know from experience, the more we know that change is possible. We must remind the client to acknowledge all changes, however slight, because each change leads to another and each slight change is progress.

When we teach from experience, we are in a better position to help the client learn without judgment. We also teach in such a manner that the person cannot fail because realistic goals are developed that can be measured. For example, a person with heart disease should be encouraged to "be with the process," and not to blame himself or herself for the symptoms of heart disease, but to know for example, that the pain medication is in the body and working as breathing and imagery exercises are used to decrease the person's chest pain and anxiety. The individual must be reminded that the body is not the problem but part of the solution.

As we teach clients to reframe experiences positively their internal thoughts are very changeable. Clients are then more able to create new beliefs that most often lead to new, healthier response patterns. If failure is not reframed it leads to more failure. Instead of the saying "the glass is half empty," reframe it by saying "the glass is half full." We must also encourage the client to involve friends and family in the learning. Learning is an ongoing process and new skills must be practiced, shared, and integrated into all aspects of life.

REFERENCES

Achterberg, J. (1990). *Women as healer.* Boston, MA: Shambhala Publications, Inc.

Achterberg, J., Dossey, B., & Kolkmeier, L. (1994). *Rituals of healing.* New York: Bantam Books.

Barnsteiner, J., Gillis-Donovan, J., Knox-Fischer, C., & McKlindon, D. (1994). Defining and implementing a standard for therapeutic relationships. *Journal of Holistic Nursing, 12* (1), 35–49.

Benner, P., & Wrubel, J. (1989). *The primacy of caring.* Menlo Park, CA: Addison-Wesley Publishing Company.

Burkhardt, M., & Nagai-Jacobson, M. G. (1994). Reawakening spirit in clinical practice. *Journal of Holistic Nursing 12* (1), 9–21.

Burkhardt, M. (1989). Spirituality: An analysis of the concept. *Holistic Nursing Practice, 3* (3), 69–77.

Carper, B. (1978). Fundamental patterns of knowing. *Advances in Nursing Science, 1* (1), 13–23.

Clark, C., & Heidenreich, T. (1995). Spiritual care for the critically ill. *American Journal of Critical Care, 4* (1), 77.

Dossey, B. (1995a). The psychophysiology of bodymind healing. In Dossey, B., Keegan, L., Guzzetta, C., & Kolkmeier, L., *Holistic nursing: A handbook for practice* (2nd ed.). Gaithersburg, MD: Aspen Publishers, Inc.

Dossey, B., & Guzzetta, C. (1995b). Holistic nursing practice. In Dossey, B., Keegan, L., Guzzetta, C., & Kolkmeier, L., *Holistic nursing: A handbook for practice* (2nd ed.). Gaithersburg, MD: Aspen Publishers, Inc.

Dossey, B. (1995c). Nurse as healer. In Dossey, B., Keegan, L., Guzzetta, C., & Kolkmeier, L., *Holistic nursing: A handbook for practice* (2nd ed.). Gaithersburg, MD: Aspen Publishers, Inc.

Dracup, K., & Bryan-Brown, W. (1995). Humane care in inhumane places. *American Journal of Critical Care, 4* (1), 1.

Gilje, F. (1992). Being there: An analysis of the concept of presence. In Gaut, D. (Ed.), *The presence of caring in nursing.* New York: National League for Nursing Press.

Harvey, M. A. (1994). An era of opportunity. *American Journal of Critical Care, 3* (4), 320. President's Commission for the Study of Ethical Problems in Medicine and Biomedical and Behavioral Research. *Deciding to forego life sustaining treatment.* Washington, DC: US Government Printing Office, *5* (1),17.

Hendricks, G., & Hendricks, K. *At the speed of life.* New York: Bantam Books.

Karl, J. (1992). Being there: Who do you bring to practice. In Gaut, D. (Ed.), *The presence of caring in nursing.* New York: National League for Nursing Press.

Keegan L. (1994). *Nurse as healer.* New York: Delmar Publishers, Inc.

Mayeroff, M. (1972). *On caring.* New York: Harper & Row.

McKivergin, M. (1994). The essence of therapeutic presence. *Journal of Holistic Nursing, 12* (1), 65–81.

Montgomery, C. (1992). The spiritual connection: Nurses' perceptions of the experience of caring. In Gaut, D. (Ed.), *The presence of caring in nursing.* New York: National League for Nursing Press.

Morse, J., et al. (1991). Comparative analysis of conceptualizations and theories of caring. *Image, 23* (2), 119–126.

Munhall, P. (1993). Unknowing: Toward another pattern of knowing in nursing. *Nursing Outlook, 41* (1), 125–128.

Newman, M. (1994). *Health as expanding consciousness.* New York: National League for Nursing Press.

Patient Rights: Accreditation manual for hospitals. (1992). Chicago, IL, Joint Commission on Accreditation of Healthcare Organizations (suppl).

Peper, E., & Kuskel, C. (1985). A holistic merger of biofeedback and family therapy. In Kunz, D., (Ed.), *Spiritual aspects of the healing arts.* Wheaton,IL: The Theosophical Publishing House.

Remen, R. (1993). The eye of an eagle, the heart of a lion, the hand of a woman, *The Journal of the Healing Health Care Project 2* (3), 16–19.

Roach, M. S. (1987). *The human act of caring.* Ottawa: Canadian Hospital Association.

Watson, J. (1988). *Nursing: Human science and human care.* New York: National League for Nursing Press.

Wolfer, J. (1993). Aspects of reality and ways of knowing in nursing: In search of an integrating paradigm. *Image 2* (2), 141–145.

PROFILES
OF NURSE
HEALERS

SHARING OUR HEALING STORIES

Most nurses are very modest and take their healing qualities and interactions for granted. The profound healing that often takes place in the ordinariness, such as the way a nurse touches a client in taking a blood pressure or how a nurse prepares a patient for surgery and is present in the unknowing, is not often valued or even recognized by the nurse as healing moments. Do you have trouble talking about healing and what you do as a nurse to facilitate healing? Nurses can learn to become open and comfortable in talking about healing. Some comments by nurses are, "Well that is what I do because I am a nurse," or "It is expected that I help clients." Frequently, nurses do not give themselves credit for healing moments and this leads to burnout and the expression "Same old thing, day-in and day-out." When was the last time that you created time within yourself to affirm the value of your actions and your presence with yourself or another? Can you recall saying to yourself "I did a wonderful job," and then feeling inspired about your work and healing interactions.

Transformation of caring, healing, and innovative nursing practices begins with dialogue. The term *dialogue* is derived from a Greek word with *dia* meaning through and *logos* signifying *the word*. We cannot change in isolation. We must begin the dialogue that envisions, builds trust, and establishes community in the deepest sense. A healthy dialogue means that an individual does not hold a fixed position, but listens to others explore other realities. It means that we intently listen to another person's story so that we can more fully understand their belief system and values even when they may be foreign to us.

Nurse healers are active listeners and support each other in the change process. As we deepen our skills and awareness of love, respect, and trust between and among ourselves, each of us will be enriched. When we negate and criticize each other's wisdom, levels of fear are created within us. However, when we actively listen to new ways of participating, we build and enhance trust levels. Lack of trust creates fear and can paralyze our body-mind-spirit process. Trust levels can mobilize and enhance our healing journey, and we can more easily share our personal journey with another. As we share our healing journeys with each other, we can more easily begin a healthy dialogue among ourselves. As we do this we are also empowered toward creative action in our personal and professional lives.

The following nurse healer profiles help us appreciate the importance of sharing our own healing journeys with each other. These nurse healers are in independent practice, education, acute care, chronic and long term care, and administration. As we reflect on these personal stories we can more easily begin a healthy dialogue among ourselves. When we do this, we are also empowered toward creative action in our personal and professional lives.

NURSE HEALERS
IN INDEPENDENT
PRACTICE

3

INTRODUCTION

Increasing numbers of nurses are moving away from the traditional work setting. The reasons for this range from being "reengineered" out of an existing position because of agency downsizing or by the conscious decision of the nurse to leave the established agency setting and begin a compelling new career challenge. No matter what the reason that initiated the change, most nurses in independent practice are pioneers and pacesetters.

As we gathered our profiles, we found a number of the individuals we chose to feature are in unique practice settings. However, as you read their stories, realize that all of them have practiced in acute and chronic care settings for at least some time during their developmental years. We are certain that you will follow with interest their progression from traditional to nontraditional setting as they evolved through personal transformative experiences to arrive in their most innovative current practice settings.

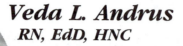

Veda L. Andrus
RN, EdD, HNC

*Program Director, AHNA Certificate
Program in Holistic Nursing
Whately, Massachusetts*

Listening to my inner voice and moving with what I hear is the most profound affirmation of my spiritual path. There will always be a wide array of voices that command attention. My personal and professional journey is about remembering my purpose and vision . . . and allowing all the other voices and energies to proceed on their journeys as well.

I recall, as if it were yesterday, filling out college applications to major in music. I was never the least bit interested in becoming a nurse. The Future Nurses Club at my high school in Pough-keepsie, New York, did not draw my attention. I was an accomplished pianist and saw music as a creative expression and my future career. I had the college applications filled out with music as my declared major when at the eleventh hour, I literally crossed out music and wrote in nursing. I cannot tell you where this came from at the time. Now as I reflect, I deeply understand this as divine guidance and am grateful for having listened and responded.

Upon receiving a BSN degree from the University of Miami in 1973, I went directly into an MSN program at the University of Arizona where my specialty was as a generalist in clinical practice. Although this predated Nurse Practitioner programs, it achieved the same goal of providing direct patient care within a clinical setting. In 1975, I moved to Connecticut to accept a position as a nurse practitioner at the Wesleyan University Student Health Services. By my second year there, I realized that I no longer believed in the type of health care I was providing. I began to talk about attitudes and beliefs regarding health and healing and drove students to the health food store while discussing nutrition, stress management, and self-care. I realized I no longer came from my heart within my nursing practice and, hence, left the nursing profession in 1977.

The years from 1977 until 1983 were years of searching for my self. I worked in natural food stores and food co-ops to financially support myself as I moved to Boston and later to Portland, Oregon; Santa Fe, New Mexico; and finally, thirteen years ago, to what is now my home in western Massachusetts. I kept my nursing license active in each state where I lived, but could not bring myself to practice in a health care system that did not resonate with my spirit. I suppose one could say that my primary obstacle at this time was my heart! Although these were challenging and confusing times, in retrospect, I have a deep respect for my choice of listening to my truth and by not practicing nursing in a manner that was incongruent with my heartfull knowing.

Three days after I moved to Massachusetts in 1983, I was handed a catalog from the Omega Institute for Holistic Studies announcing a weekend workshop called "Nurses in Transition." There was no question in my mind that I was, indeed, a nurse in transition! I attended the workshop along with forty-five other nurses of like mind and vision, knowing I had come home to the heart and spirit of nursing.

For the following two years, I co-taught a five-day workshop at Omega called "New Directions in Nursing." In 1985, Charlotte McGuire, founder of the American Holistic Nurses' Association (AHNA), presented a keynote address for our workshop and later asked me to serve as Northeast Regional Director for the Association. I wasn't even a member of AHNA yet! I agreed to serve in the position, quickly joined AHNA, and have been passionately committed to the vision and practice of holistic nursing ever since.

I was a novice in holistic nursing and felt rather uncertain about myself in this new position as a leader. While at a Board of Directors meeting in Telluride, Colorado, a well-seasoned board member raised the idea that the AHNA needed to develop a certificate Program in Holistic Nursing and asked if someone on the Board would be willing to initiate and direct this process. In what I now (ten years later) affectionately call an "out-of-body experience," my hand shot up, volunteering for what has become a remarkable journey of personal, mutual, universal transformation and healing.

I was fortunate to access a small group of holistically minded nurses in my community and invited them to co-participate in the creation of what is now the internationally recognized AHNA Certificate Program in Holistic Nursing. I continue to serve as the

Program Director and am currently teaching and expanding the program with my business partner and colleague, Jane Yetter Lunt. This innovative and integrative program is presented in a dynamic way to provide nurses with a foundation of holistic philosophy and holistic nursing theory in which to ground their nursing practice. I will not share all the details of its development; suffice it to say that this has been and continues to be a journey of conscious intention heartfelt passion, and commitment to assist in the evolution of the current health care system into one of caring by, for, and about ourselves, other beings, our planet, and the broader universe.

I view the AHNA Certificate Program in Holistic Nursing as an opportunity for professional development through which nurses are encouraged to empower themselves with new ways of being so they are as present, available, and mindful as they would like to be with their patients/clients. They come together as a community of nurses with a common vision and return to their homes embraced within a network of professional support. Upon returning to their home environment, these nurses carry with them a message that they are bright spirits within the universe with the capacity to influence others by coming from their hearts and living in a new way.

Simultaneous to the development and teaching of the AHNA Certificate Program in Holistic Nursing, I returned to graduate school in 1991 at the University of Massachusetts and received a Doctorate in Education with a concentration in organizational development and transformational leadership. I integrated many of the concepts of this leadership ideology and incorporated them within my position as President of the American Holistic Nurses' Association. I served in this capacity until 1993 when I became the AHNA International Director. During my two year tenure as International Director, I was selected by the Citizen Ambassador Program of People to People International to serve as the delegation leader on a professional exchange program to China and Mongolia.

All the experiences of my life are integral to who I am today as a certified holistic nurse (HNC) and a human being. I believe that I am an expression of the Earth and that I am here in physical form to manifest the full creative potential of my spirit. For me, this is best done by trusting what I hear from within and moving with what I know to be my truth. Perhaps an awareness that all beings are one with the Earth will be the paradigm shift necessary for healing ourselves, all beings, and our planet.

I feel fortunate to have embarked upon a remarkable journey, one that has allowed me the opportunity to co-create a vehicle for nurses to reflect upon their presence and influence in our world. My intention has always been to be an active change agent in encouraging nurses to come from their hearts and spirits through the scientific art of nursing practice. It is my responsibility to remain clear to my purpose and vision, to honor and respect the diversity of nurses who touch my life, and to do so mindfully and with integrity.

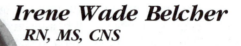

Irene Wade Belcher
RN, MS, CNS

Senior Editor, AHNA, Beginnings Newsletter
Tucker, Georgia

Somewhere deep within, I have always sensed that healing into, or rediscovering, our own wholeness is what each of our human journeys is really all about. My birth occurred at what might be described as the best and the worst of times. World War II had just ended, and in 1946, along with the first crop of babyboomers, I made my not-so-grand entrance, one filled with tremendous fear and trepidation. Not wanting to face life as on a soul level I knew it to be, I literally came through the birth process without my mother's water breaking, presenting with a "veil" over my face. The corner of the world I entered, the rural South, was one filled with poverty, struggle for survival, and racial intensity, and my lessons early on were those of learning to cope and survive in an impoverished and unloving world.

Upon completion of high school, my heartfelt desire was to study journalism. I wanted to write. About what, I'm not sure. I just knew that journalism, like a magnet, drew me. However, in those days professional choices for women were essentially limited to the big three: secretary, teacher, or nurse. The natural career choice for me appeared to be nursing. I emphasize natural because I had spent my life caretaking an emotionally dependent, deaf mother, and an emotionally and mentally dysfunctional father.

Nursing school proved invaluable. It was through nursing that I perceived a part of myself I later identified as the unhealthy caretaker. Experiences in the years that followed continued to mirror to me who I was in relationship to that role. I chose career paths that revealed healthier ways to care for myself and others. Those career choices, in conjunction with many hours of private therapy, greatly enhanced my personal growth.

In the early 1980s, I opened a private practice as a Rehabilitation Consultant. For eight years I worked with clients who were in chronic pain due to severe injuries, illness, or both. These wonderful teachers provided me with daily, in-depth lessons about the true courage and determination it takes for one to heal.

Years later, I would draw heavily on those memories when I found myself desperately seeking my own way back to wholeness.

With my marriage in 1984 came the luxury of pursuing other career interests. Counseling at a psychiatric chronic pain clinic was a welcome new venture. Impressed with the positive effects of hypnosis, meditation, and interactive guided imagery on chronic pain, I became a proficient practitioner of those modalities gaining certification as a professional hypnotherapist.

The study and practice of hypnotherapy opened another door—one that was unexpected and in no way consciously pursued. The safe place I had secured in my marriage combined with continuous exposure to trance states set the stage for the awakening of my inner healer.

My personal time of healing was also an intense time of learning, about spirituality, faith, trust, surrender, letting go, flowing with the process. I had to be frequently reminded to "trust the process." Forced to live in the moment, my journey became truly transformational. It was during this "shaman's" journey that I came to fully understand that conventional medicine did not begin to have total answers for, or meet the needs of, others like myself, who were experiencing phenomena that were far beyond western medicine's ability to explain, let alone treat.

Books and literature that needed to come my way indeed began "falling off the shelves." Somewhere in the throes of that difficult process, there came a "knowing" that when I was well enough, my life's mission would be that of spreading holism—the concept of healing the whole person—mind, body, soul, and spirit. I knew my life's work was to be that of establishing channels through which holism could be communicated.

In 1989, I returned to full-time work as a Home Health Liaison Consultant. For two and a half years I continued to hang somewhere between fragility and functionality—my spirit was more than willing, but my physical and emotional energies were not yet strong enough for me to embrace my vision. By 1992, I felt I could take on school. On entering a Masters Program in Psychiatric Nursing, my dream began to take form. Still, it was not enough. Shortly after beginning that program, my hunger to be with and learn from others who were of like-mind led me to found the Atlanta Holistic Nurses' Network. At that time my husband, David, helped me to secure my long time dream of

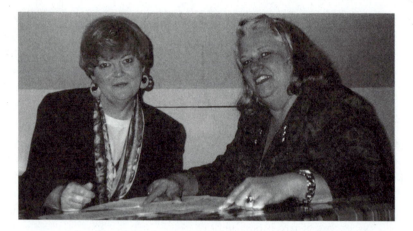

becoming a journalist. Together, we began publishing a local newsletter, *HoloGram*. Within 3 years our network mushroomed from 200 to 800 people.

The year 1995 marked a time of an outflowing of blessings from the Universe. On completion of my graduate program, Sigma Theta Tau honored me with the Highest Graduate Achievement Award, recognizing my accomplishments in the promotion of holistic nursing and mind-body medicine. That same year the American Holistic Nurses' Association asked that I become the Senior Editor of their national newsletter, *Beginnings*. I was further honored with an appointment to the National Leadership Council of AHNA.

I am privileged to have been given the opportunity to practice my other love—teaching student nurses. My message to all nurses, students or otherwise, can be found in my philosophy of nursing which also translates into my life's philosophy: As part of the human condition, we are constantly being challenged to heal into more wholeness. How much we choose to heal is a decision that we, as responsible individuals, must make.

My core premise regarding illness of any kind is that, for the most part, it originates from disharmony between different aspects of one's perceived "self." As human beings we are constantly being offered opportunities to transform belief patterns that create distress on mental, emotional, physical, and spiritual levels. As a nurse, I choose to educate clients about choices of when and how they might heal. I also choose to empower them by reminding them of their inherent ability to self-heal, but I have come to understand over the years how important it is that I not take on another's heal-ing process. This kind of expanded consciousness leads to a more total honoring of both self and others which, to me, is the hallmark of a healthy interconnectedness of body, mind, soul, and spirit. Recognizing and honoring each person's individual, unique, and chosen place in his or her own human experience defines the boundaries within which I function in my roles as a human being, as an educator, and as a professional nurse.

Finally, I perceive that every person I encounter brings back to me a part of myself that was missing. When that part resonates within, it is transformative, drawing me closer to my own whole-ness. Such experiences over time have confirmed to me that heal-ing seldom, if ever, involves or affects just one person. Rather, we are all continually, knowingly or unknowingly, participating together as co-partners in healing.

Mary J. Frost
RN, MS, CHTP/I

Co-founder and Educational Director,
Total Health, Inc., Holistic Nursing
Associates and Consultants
Covington, Louisiana

I was born in the post World War II years in the American Midwest in Coldwater, Michigan, a small town that served as a last stop for the Underground Railroad during the Civil War days. Many of the large, old homes there had secret rooms and passageways in which to sequester runaway slaves who came North coveting their freedom. At that time my father was an intern at the local community hospital and my mother had left her career as a hospital dietitian to raise the children. Both had served in the army during the war, in fact they met while at boot camp. My mother was the daughter of a poor dust bowl farmer and a strong German wife who went west in the Oklahoma land rush in the late 1800s. My paternal grandfather was a large animal veterinarian and professor of veterinary medicine. My paternal grandmother was a nurse. She bequeathed to me her brass teapot and candle-powered warmer that she used during her nursing years.

Another very influential part of my family heritage was the strong sense of service that I witnessed during my childhood. My parents were committed to sharing and caring for everyone who appeared in their lives. We always had extra children in our home and even took them on vacation trips. Every holiday and many Sundays we had at least one foreign college student included in the festivities, and during the winter my mother collected coats and other warm clothing for the ones who came to study in Michigan from the tropics. During my high school years I was part of an ecumenical church youth group that was involved in a great deal of service work. I can remember painting a church to house a migrant Mexican congregation, helping to renovate a house for a VISTA volunteer on a local American Indian reservation, and going into the locked ward of a state mental institution to visit the patients and act as envoys from the outside world. We would manicure and paint the women's fingernails and simply sit and talk with them one on one. I enjoyed all of these activities. There was a knowing within me that I would continue to find ways to serve others.

After high school I made several attempts at college, but it got in the way of seeing the world. Many years were spent on domestic and foreign travel and working various jobs. On one occasion, I traveled to Europe for a summer college semester and discovered the challenge of mountain climbing. Then I traveled and climbed; the pièce de résistance was the Matterhorn in Zermatt, Switzerland, which was my ultimate challenge. I was satisfied that I could live and travel in foreign countries and climb perilous peaks, but I was always pulled back at quiet times when I was alone to an inner discontent. What was this nameless yearning that called to me from inside? I would listen for awhile, make an attempt to quiet it by working with emotionally disturbed children, or in the inner city schools, or tutor illiterate adults. But distractions came and I was off following another rainbow.

Finally when I was in my mid-thirties, domestication swooned over my life and I married and had my son. I focused on important issues. I realized how much it meant to me to have a nurse-midwife attend to my prenatal, postnatal, and birth experience. I became dedicated to saving this sacred experience for women and actively supported the licensing of midwives in my state. I used herbs to treat myself for minor health imbalances and actively participated in a natural foods cooperative. My diet became basically vegetarian and my food staple was organic brown rice. I exercised and taught aerobics. I needed a forum to learn and to share what I was experiencing in my life.

When I returned to college, this time with an infant son, I was determined to feed my internal soul demands. I switched my majors from psychology and French to pre-physical therapy. Obstacles kept appearing, but finally I gave up resistance and went through the open door that appeared, nursing. I had come home. Finally, my first paper was on holistic health care, as this philosophy was truly believable, livable, and practical. My father, the physician, had told me that one of the most powerful medicines was, "tincture of time," in that many maladies had a way of disappearing on their own. Sometimes the best intervention was

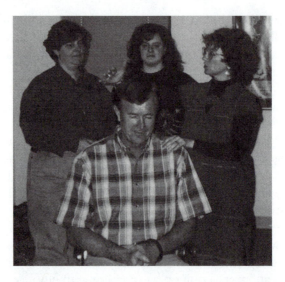

no intervention. My mother had shown me that acceptance of another, no matter the circumstance, was the best place to start giving love.

So I graduated cum laude with a baccalaureate degree in nursing at 40, having passed through the "hoops of fire," to begin nursing in a holistic way. How was I going to do that with no immediate role models? Where were the people that I had read about in the books and journals? I found them upon graduation at the AHNA Annual Conference in Green Lake, Wisconsin. I entered a room back of the conference room after having driven for two solid days with upper back and neck pain from physical stress. I was awestruck. The room was filled with so much light from radiant beings who hugged one another with love in their eyes. There was support without competitiveness. There was possibility without question. There was hope without fear. I was literally shown the way by these healed nurses who were living examples of joyful empowerment. I felt so small and weak. These nurses reached out to me. One of them gave me the gift of her friendship. Another helped me to cry. Yet another laid her hands on my back and neck until I deeply relaxed and the tension and pain went away.

I knew after 40 years what my inner voice was trying to tell me, why I always felt a discontent in the quiet after fervent activity. The spirit of both of my grandmothers was alive in me, the nurse caregiver and the pioneer driving fast into unknown territory. I would become healed too, and in the process would understand how to help others go through that process, whatever it was. I would follow my internal voice and direction.

Things happened fast after attending that conference, and automatically and easily. Soon I had signed up for a Healing Touch workshop and convinced a nurse friend to go along. We traveled around the country until we had completed the program. We were in the historical first group to apply for Healing Touch Certification quickly followed by the instructor certification. My full-time job at the hospital gave way to work at a general practice clinic, then to independent practice. Now I am doing what makes my heart sing. I work with clients, seeing them for Healing Touch energy work and hypnotherapy, which is integrated with a wide variety of other complementary modalities such as guided imagery, aromatherapy, healing sound and music, attentive listening, and whatever else it seems the client needs. Mostly I act as a mirror, in which I reflect to clients their own light and life patterns, so they can gain insight into how to love themselves and move toward healthier patterns, and let their own light shine. It is joyful work and takes me into the public school system, the hospital, a person's home, or wherever I am called. Much of my time is spent talking to groups, professional nurses, support groups, public forums, and in teaching classes in energy healing to nurses, massage therapy students, and the interested public.

Being a healer is being healed and holding the space so that others may be healed. It is an evolving process and a deepening process, learning to listen to the messages from the body, heart, mind, and soul and from the universal intelligence that exists in all things. It is remembering to pay attention to the beauty of the sunset or the longing of another human, and being truly present for every precious moment.

Dorothea Hover-Kramer
RN, EdD, CHTP/I

Licensed Clinical Psychologist and Director
Behavioral Health Consultants
Poway, California

I was born in Berlin, Germany, exactly nine months after the big war, World War II, started in Europe. I was the only one in the family who never knew what life was like without war since I was the youngest child of two well-known German scientists and had four bossy older siblings. My grandmother, the wife of a loving physician, was my favorite person. She seemed to understand me and tried to explain why things were burning and being destroyed around us. She fell off a bridge when I was a little over two years old. I distinctly remember searching for her, and when I found her, trying to make her feel better. She never recovered mentally or physically, deteriorating over several years. Her absence without actual death became my first experience of inconsolable loss, of confronting forces beyond my own capacity.

By the time I was five, I was basically a war orphan although my older siblings tried their best to offset the incredible losses and destruction of saturation bombing. Two glimpses of pleasure came into my life. After the invasion of Berlin by the allies, an American soldier came to the yard and gave me a black doll, a colored version of Raggedy Ann. Someone explained that no one wanted this doll because it was black. I scooped her up and decided to give her my finest care, although I was ridiculed a good bit by my elders for having such an unusual "doll child".

The other glimpse of joy was in taking care of birds. The big shade trees in our neighborhood were being cut for firewood because there was no other fuel. A refugee brought in a nest full of half-grown fledglings. I had no idea what to feed them but saved some of my bread crusts for them. The other thing I could do was to hold them in my hands and warm them. Then I discovered I could simply hold my hands over the birds that were too jittery to be picked up. Soon, other neighbors were bringing me birds of all sizes since the adults admitted they just did not have time for such trivia. Bringing my full intent and prayers to these little ones taught me some valuable lessons: one, I learned how much I yearned to make our disrupted environment better; another, that some birds actually got better and could fly away after a few days; and finally that some birds apparently could not live and died. My sister and I staged elaborate funeral ceremonies, an activity that seemed appropriate with all the loss and dying happening all around. To this day, I am honored that animals seem to be comfortable with me. I have many pets and live in a wilderness area where hawks and coyotes abound, east of San Diego.

My family emigrated to the United States before I was ten to join my father, a scientist who had been selected by the American Navy just after the war to continue his research in silicate sciences. I never thought much about nursing until I had graduated from high school and found music school much too confining. The family was disappointed that I did not want to be a professional musician, and I was told there were no funds for other college programs, unless, of course, I wanted to go to medical school and make something important of myself. Instead, I enrolled in a diploma nursing program at Flower Hospital in Toledo Ohio, a program I could easily afford. I fully expected to learn all about healing as I had read in Florence Nightingale's books.

My teachers tried to assure me that I was learning how to help people with all the medications and treatment protocols we studied. My heart told me otherwise. Somehow, we should be able to do things more directly, it seemed to me, without waiting for a doctor's order. I kept thinking nurses should be more independent and authoritative, and I disagreed regularly with my instructors.

Nevertheless I graduated with top honors and decided to get my bachelor's degree in nursing at Boston University. Again the dilemma, we learned many fine concepts, but nothing about hands-on healing. I decided to try public health and home care. Some of the elderly patients I visited had severe decubiti with poor potential for wound closure. I put my hands over the area after doing dressing changes, adding the fervent prayers I had used with the little birds. My patients told me how warm my hands felt although I was not touching them. In two to four weeks these deep ulcers healed over, quite beyond my own expectations. Even now, I am always surprised when something actually changes as I set my focused intent for healing in whatever way is needed.

As a diligent public health nurse with a master's degree, I tried to approach physical healing from an epidemiological framework. I saw the interconnections between a person's thinking patterns, emotional states, and the onset of physical illness. Could severe illness be prevented if we worked with the emotions during or after a stressful event or loss? It made sense that primary prevention would be better than intervening after the onset of disease, so I studied psychology, and completed my doctorate in 1978. By then, I had already started a private practice of psychotherapy and began to specialize in working with bereavement and chronic pain.

The advent of the American Holistic Nurses' Association (AHNA) gave me a conceptual framework for the multidimensional processes involved in genuine healing. It was exciting to meet fellow professionals who, like myself, were seeking integrative pathways to healing by focusing on the whole person, mind and emotions, body and spirit. I served seven years as a board member of the AHNA, and was involved in laying the groundwork of the Holistic Nursing and Healing Touch certification programs, which have now become large, recognized programs in holism.

Throughout the last twenty years, I have seen clients with complex body and mind problems, such as cancer, AIDS, environmental illnesses, Chronic Fatigue Syndrome, as well as more pervasive psychological problems, like depression and anxiety. About fifteen years ago, I started using my hands in my clients' energy fields, above their physical bodies, to facilitate deep relaxation and clear out tension. The results were always similar—relief of anxiety, release of muscle tension, deeper breathing and relaxation, and an enhanced sense of well-being. As a scientist, I paid attention to these phenomena and started reading all I could to support my actions. As an artist, I began enjoying the creativity of going beyond verbal therapy to deeper states of subconscious awareness.

Over time, through many challenges in my family life, I have become more skilled, not only in tracing my own spiritual journey but in assisting others to find their transpersonal connections. I have learned to trust my intuition as well as my knowledge base and to recognize that every client brings me a gift—the gift of trust, the gift of wanting to have a fuller life even when there is incurable illness, the gift of unique willingness to try out a new approach.

My greatest obstacles have been my own lack of trust, lack of hope, and lack of resourcefulness in getting help for myself. While I can look at external obstacles, such as loss of loved ones, pain, and divorce with some candor, there is always a personal shadow part that remains hidden, outside of my awareness. Like the proverbial blind spot when one is driving a car, I have learned to assume that there is an area I cannot see, a part I might be missing. I ask a lot of questions now. I never send letters on the day I write them but try to think of all the ways that something might be viewed by another person. I call my friends regularly to get feedback. I journal, keep track of my dreams, and read Tarot cards weekly. If I have emotional pain for more than a day, I call one of my therapists. If I have physical distress, I get it checked out quickly, and I have body work for maintenance every other week. I see self-care as the central core of my healership journey so I can be a compassionate presence to others. I still have distress, just as my clients do. I just don't keep it for very long.

Ruth L. Johnson
RN, PhD

Co-Founder and Director, HAPPEN
Black Mountain, North Carolina

I was born in Lincoln, Nebraska, a few months after a major life-style change for the family. My parents, expecting their tenth child, moved the family from an Antelope county farm to Lincoln to take advantage of a better school system, and to have access to the university.

My early years provided a strong orientation to group process and to entrepreneurship. Everyone was encouraged to participate in creative problem solving to make this new life style as successful as possible. Five paper routes, baby sitting, establishing a lunchroom in the living/dining area of the home, alterations, and gardening on a large scale were some of the solutions. Each of us children earned enough money to make it possible; we were taught to open first a savings account, and then a checking account, as "business" needs warranted. Each child was helped to learn to manage individual finances, and each contributed to the group, both in money and in effort.

I don't recall exactly when I decided to be a nurse. It was an early interest, partly stimulated by my aunt, and deepened by the experiences during my father's lingering illness and death from Hodgkin's disease when I was sixteen. I chose the university nursing program, completing two years of pre-nursing on the Lincoln campus, then completing the five-year program with a baccalaureate degree on the Omaha campus—the Colleges of Medicine and Nursing are in Omaha. My major interest was in psychiatric nursing; we were fortunate to have a progressive program, and a psychiatric unit in the university hospital.

After working in psychiatric nursing for several years, I received my masters degree in psychiatric nursing from the University of Nebraska in 1956. I chose this program because of the strong leadership of Theresa G. Muller, RN, MA, who came to Nebraska after establishing four other masters' programs in psychiatric nursing. She had been instrumental in obtaining recognition for nursing as one of the four major disciplines in mental health, and in securing stipends for graduate study in the field. Theresa provided another major learning experience in entrepreneurship.

My nursing career involved a combination of clinical and academic work, with teaching a prominent part of each position. The settings varied from the university to heading a program in a general hospital, providing educational experiences for undergraduates within state hospitals, community mental health centers, and back to another university setting. I received my doctorate in nursing, with a minor in sociology, from Wayne State University in psychotherapy.

I don't think I ever considered myself a "healer" (my emphasis was more on "caring") until my bout with cancer. However, I was always holistically inclined and clinically oriented, maintaining focus on mind-body-spirit when many of my colleagues were focused specifically on psychotherapy.

I was trying to maintain my sanity in an academic setting while teaching, maintaining a clinical practice, and doing research all at the same time. In the unrealistic expectation of academia it was required that nurses do all of these activities, and of course publish, as well. I survived it until I took on some administration in addition, and that's when my system broke down. My last position was as Director of the Graduate Program in Nursing at Rutgers, the State University of New Jersey. By June of 1986 I was very stressed from the job, my mother's recent death, my housemate's long battle with cancer and her death. I left New Jersey and moved to Oregon with the intention of taking a reasonable vacation to heal and make future decisions.

Six months later I was diagnosed with breast cancer. I decided that an early retirement, and not a return to nursing, would enhance my survival. I am basically Rogerian in approach and believe that cancer is a response to stress which compromises the immune system. In my selection of treatment, I was guided by that premise: do everything I could to enhance immune function, and nothing that would suppress immune response. Thus, I opted for a modified radical mastectomy, and refused both chemotherapy and radiation, even though there was extensive node involvement. Confronted with the promise by the oncologist that I wouldn't live two years without chemotherapy, I embarked upon a search of alternative modalities. The literature was just beginning,

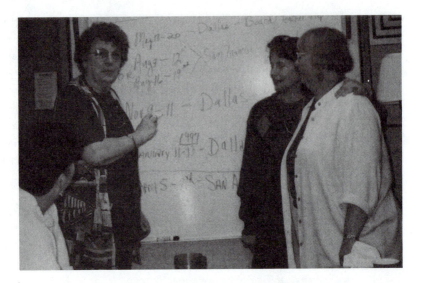

and I started off with some of Louise Hay's work, traveled to meet some of the known healers, learned about vitamin therapy and other approaches. I went to Wichita for a conference and met Dorothea Hover-Kramer, who introduced me to the American Holistic Nurses' Association and the Healing Touch Program.

Thus began my second career. I came out of retirement, joined the AHNA, and completed the Healing Touch (HT) Program, including teacher preparation. I came to HT with a theoretical background in Martha Rogers' and Dolores Krieger's work, but without the clinical experience. I then established a practice in energetic therapy, combining it with counseling. The struggle to trust my intuition in the arena of individual, group, and family psychotherapy laid the foundation for recognizing intuition as my strongest asset in energetic healing.

I think my current commitment to holistic nursing is best expressed through a new organization that I helped to establish, the Holistic Alliance for Professional Practitioners, Entrepreneurs and Networkers, Inc. (HAPPEN). Although occasionally I think about retirement, I get the message that my current role is to facilitate interaction among these dynamic, high-powered nursing leaders. This challenge calls for all the skills I have developed in prior settings.

HAPPEN is currently engaged in the development of a program to prepare "Transformational Healers" in the use of a broad range of alternative modalities, with a major emphasis on facilitating self-help. I believe this competency-based program will fill a need for those individuals who are struggling to bridge right-brain/left-brain and Eastern/Western philosophies of health care. The group picture I'm shown in here was taken at a HAPPEN meeting. We are an interesting group, with all leaders and no followers. It is our aim to set the climate that allows us to tap all of the healing skills of the group members in the work of the organization as well as in the clinical practice of its members.

I think the most important message I have to share with other healers is to deal with your own issues. We are more successful in helping others if we model the holistic process toward wellness. This requires dealing with the issues, blind spots, and unresolved conflicts that exist for all of us. A major part of this is in learning to value ourselves. I also encourage others to maintain a healthy skepticism, but remain open to ideas that may not make any sense to you at first. There are many available solutions to our problems if we can expand our views of the world sufficiently to allow us to become aware of them.

Maggie McKivergin
RN, MS

Life Coach/Consultant
Columbus, Ohio

I was born in Ft. Wayne, Indiana, on March 22, 1953. I reflect the ancestry of hard working Irish Catholic farmers which is spiced with a bit of the blarney and a love of nature, God and others. My Irish heritage helps me connect with others in loving and heart-centered ways and lightens up the cloudiest of days.

My German ancestry is most represented by my paternal great-grandfather who was a jeweler and whose precision and ability for efficiency, timing, and analysis of a system have contributed to my ability to manifest those qualities.

Music, dance, and nature are stabilizing forces in my life that have been carried down from both sides of my family. The gift of whimsical whistles through the rhythm of get-down drumming has added to my holy sound. I enjoy toning in places where sound can resonate within and around the environment and heal my being . . . my favorite place being the hills of West Virginia. I believe rhythm and resonance are integrating forces within our lives and within the relationship we have with ourselves, others, nature, and our Creator. I continue to learn about the rhythm of life and my response to its flow, leading me to the essence of my being.

I happened into nursing in 1972 with a simple desire to help others. By coincidence, I was accepted into St. Mary's School of Nursing in Huntington, West Virginia. I specialized in critical care and on two separate occasions in my career, I became burned out, losing my ability to care for others.

These were turning points in my understanding of two key ingredients to nursing: the importance of looking at the person as a whole and the importance of taking care of myself. I began to look beyond the patients' disease, recognizing the important of life events and significant relationships upon their health. It was then that human nature became a fascination to me and the mystery of life unfolding was the most intriguing ever.

Since that time, I have encountered the depths of the human condition, experiencing people's pain, confusion, abandonment, and closure as a result of their interpretation of life's experiences. I have been on a personal journey towards truth and continue to be shaped by the uniqueness of my path. My nursing background has brought me the skills and appreciation of the miracle of life, the transcendence of death and the preciousness of the human spirit. For this, I am truly grateful for it has brought a depth to the meaning and purpose of life.

In nursing school, I was on a retreat in which I experienced the presence of God, opening up to universal love and truth. The message I carry forward from that experience is one of love: for our Creator, each other, creation, and ourselves. I believe the essence of disease is rooted in a separateness or block to the flow of love in any of those dimensions and the key to healing is in connecting and becoming whole in our essence of love.

I believe I am an instrument of God's love and in keeping aligned with God's love flowing through me and energized by nature, loving friends, and family and connectedness to my personal healing, create a field that attracts people. This field is like a magnet, bringing forth others' concerns, worries, and pain and in a loving response, helps others to love themselves, others, Creator, and creation.

What I have learned as a nurse is a study of the essence of life—that which affects our spirit, our heart and emotions, our

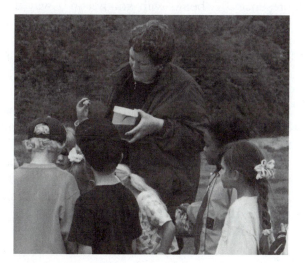

physical response to our perceptions of life's events, our relationships with self and others, our alignment with the expression of
who we are in our vocation and creative response to life.

I now have a private practice in which I nurture the identity,
purpose, health, and wholeness of others and help them to determine their direction in life. I compliment this process of inner
work through healing prayer, healing touch, Bach flowers, aromas
and magnetic therapy to balance the individual. In addition, three
precious partners and I are working to create a center for lifelong
learning and healing which will support individuals, families,
schools, churches, corporations, and communities in their search
for well-being.

In being present to my own health, I have a wonderful team
of people who nurture me and are instruments in my ongoing
process of healing. They heal by offering their gifts in unconditional love, mirroring to me my potential and encouraging me to
step forward into becoming light. Included in this team are my
wellness coach, homeopathic physician, chiropractor, applied
kinesthesiologist, rolfer, massage therapist, counselor, spiritual
director, healing touch practitioner, reflexologist, and my dear
friends and family.

I am thankful for all that has been given to me and hope to
keep open in a flow of giving and receiving life in love. My evolution as a nurse has led me from acquiring the skills and talents
for safe and effective practice to studying the art of therapeutic
presence . . . being with another in a way that will affect their
healing. To me, nurturing the human spirit is in listening to the
story of each individual and journeying with another in the person's walk through life. The partnership and gift of presence that
I offered during this time allows another the security to explore
and open up to new possibilities for life.

I have faith in the future, in direct relationship with how we
bring our truth, hope, love, integrity, respect, care and of presence
to ourselves, each other, and our children. I believe in the power
of creating community between us . . . of people who are committed to enhancing their potential as instruments of healing. The
beautiful compliment of our gifts as well as our intentions to be
light and love in the world creates the energy to transform not
only individuals but life on earth as well. Peace to all.

Susan Morales
RN, MSN, CHTP/I

Director, Healing Touch Canada, Inc., President, Canadian Healing Touch Foundation Toronto, Ontario, Canada

At first it was difficult to call myself a "nurse healer." It required time and sometimes painful steps to arrive at the place of naming myself. I explored the meaning of nursing for me and questioned, what was a healer?

It was easy to call myself a nurse. I graduated with a BSN in 1971 from the Medical College of Virginia School of Nursing. I had practiced nursing in a variety of clinical settings. I thought I knew enough about nursing to even leave it for awhile. I left it when I began to question everything in my life. During this "vision quest," my spiritual life burned with such an intensity that I was not able to see nursing as a form to support it. Nothing was more important than nurturing that spiritual hunger. At the time, I did not view nursing as "spiritual." I became a meditation teacher and taught for five years in Toronto, Canada.

"Once a nurse, always a nurse" has proven to be a true statement in my life. In teaching people to meditate, I was fascinated by their physiological improvements in health. As their ability to handle stress improved, so did their overall quality of life. I felt blessed to be able to provide people with an option for a better life. My life as well seemed to be blossoming. I had studied with an Orthodox rabbi and converted to Judaism in 1977. It felt like coming home. I married for a second time, believing in love again. Together, my husband and I created a home and a "stress management" center to teach meditation. All the while, the "nurse" inside me was watching and recording the miracles in my life as well as in those whom I taught.

I awoke after emergency surgery to find myself a patient. Pain, both physical and emotional, greeted me as the benevolent

---

Portrait photograph by Melanie Freeman

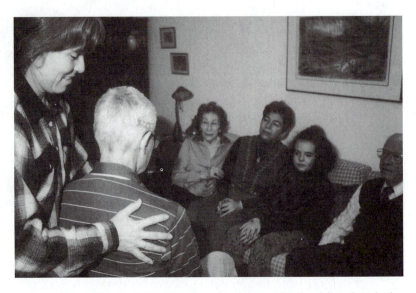

grace of anesthesia faded. I was a woman who had lost her baby and the hope of bearing children. I was a woman who no longer called herself "nurse" and was now in the hands of nurses. Vulnerable, I was keenly aware of what a nurse offered me. Was she simply "doing her job" or was she conscious of her special role in helping me heal? There were those who treated me like a piece of meat and there were others whose hands conveyed all the compassion and warmth in their hearts. It was the latter who inspired me. I remember lying in bed thinking, "I may not remember all the medications and how to calculate an IV drip, but I sure as heck can care and demonstrate that caring."

Coinciding with my return to nursing was my involvement with Therapeutic Touch (TT). In 1980 I studied with Dora Kunz and the next year with Dolores Krieger. I have continued to study with and help them each year. TT provided me with the opportunity to see that my spiritual life could be wedded with my professional life as a nurse. It was the act of centering that was the key. Each time I centered I called the most spiritual aspect of myself to the present moment. In that moment, from that compassionate place in my heart, I offered my service as a nurse. Nursing began to look and feel very different than when I had first graduated. I began to view nursing as a healing art.

But what did I know about healing? Was it the same as being "holistic"? I knew that as I practiced TT, I was aware of the different levels of the energy field. I knew I was not separate from the movement of that energy flow. "Holistic," as I understood it, was all the parts together—body, mind, spirit. This applied to me as well as to my patients. How "well" was my mind, body, spirit?

In searching for holistic resources, I discovered the American Holistic Nurses' Association. Here was a whole community of nurses who were committed to exploring the principles of holistic nursing. I joined in 1982 and served as the International Director for five years. It is one of the highlights of my professional career to have had the honor of serving on that Leadership Council. Also on the council at the time was Janet Mentgen; her Healing Touch Certificate Program was being birthed by AHNA. I became involved then and am delighted to still be as passionately committed to the program, serving as the Director of Healing Touch Canada.

Being involved with a program that focused on "healing," I found myself drawn to examine what needed healing in me. By now I was feeling very passionate about nursing. I loved being a nurse! I still believe it is an honor to bear witness to another's vulnerability. I was dismayed to see the nursing students' enthusiasm grow less each year. I wanted to shout loudly to them, to the "burned-out" nurses who were their role models, "Hey! It doesn't have to be this way! Nursing is great if you take time to take care of YOU." I needed a loud enough voice to be heard. I went to graduate school to get a big voice. I graduated from the University of Virginia with an MSN and a bigger voice in 1988.

That bigger voice did attract attention on many levels. "Be careful of what you ask for." Consciously, my bigger voice could address the need for healing in nursing. On an unconscious level, that voice was loudly calling for more healing in my personal life. The big voice attracted a big job in Vancouver, British Columbia. It was my glorious debut as a CNS in Palliative Care and my first experience with corporate politics. I failed miserably. Within a 24-hour period, I lost both my job and my husband. I was in a city with no support networks like I had in Toronto. I was alone. I lay on my living room floor staring out the windows for hours. The only thing I could do each day was to jog. Running along the ocean seemed to be a metaphor for my life. I was running for my life.

The big voice grew silent as I journeyed into the depths of my being where shadows swallow any sound. There was never any choice about the descent; the only choice was to go kicking and screaming or to walk it and stay as alert as possible. I never fought it; somewhere in my being I knew it was the natural cycle of life and death. And something was definitely dying. Even in that dark place there is a glimmer of blessing, of Light. From that glimmer I was able to see that I was dying. Who I had thought I was as defined by relationships, job, locale had all been stripped away. I stood alone on my path. Or so I thought.

That time in my life was the most awful and the most awesome. I naively named it my "dark night of the soul," assuming we only ever needed to go through ONE of them. Looking back, it was my first such experience and therefore the impact was great. It was an "initiation" of which I had only read about in relation to "healers." In my quest for discovering more about healers and healing, I had unconsciously given permission to the universe, God, whomever, to teach me in a way that guaranteed I would apply what I learned. What better way than to alter the vessel so that the contents will be congruent?

As the vessel of me shattered, I discovered that I was not alone. There was the One who was lovingly shattering the vessel so as to free the contents which could no longer be contained in that form, much like helping a snake shed its old skin. I experienced a miracle every day for the first week following the change. At first I thought they were coincidences but then realized they were telegrams from God saying, "You OK? I'm here." It was the beginning of healing for me and a deepening of a faith that will always sustain me.

I now had a better idea of what being a "healer" entailed. Becoming a healer meant that there was a conscious choice in living one's life as process. The process of healing one's own wounds is essential before one can address them in another. In my own healing I lost a big voice but gained a softer one. With a quiet voice I am able to hear the subtle nuances in my life or in my client's energy field. When I am teaching, the softer voice speaks from my heart about the love I have for the work of Healing Touch.

When asked what I do for a living, I find it easier now to say, "I'm a nurse healer." I went through a phase of feeling exuberant and proud in calling myself a nurse healer. One day I met with an old wise rabbi. In his small office, made smaller by the mounds of books stacked beside bulging bookshelves, we exchanged questions and answers. In response to his simple and direct questions concerning my spiritual life, I answered quietly and respectfully. Then he asked what I did for a living. With exuberance, I proudly declared myself a nurse healer! He looked puzzled and then quietly asked, "Since when did they put those two together?" It was a humbling moment. I wondered what he thought or knew of nursing to ponder such a question. So now I quietly respond when asked and know that there is sometimes a need to explain. I like that because it gives me another opportunity to hear myself explain who I am.

> In the name of healing
> I search for my name.
> I find it somewhere between heal
> and ing,
> between the action and the stillness.
> It is the name of all healers,
> it is
> Love.
> –*Susan Morales*

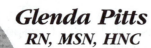
Glenda Pitts
RN, MSN, HNC

Private Practice
Louisville, Kentucky

So many lifetimes have arisen and faded since the spring of 1940 when I was born in Cincinnati, Ohio, to a couple with roots in rural southern Kentucky. Greatly treasured, and over-protected, I grew through girlhood learning the traditional values of hard work, honesty, and education. I cannot recall a time when I did not want to be a nurse. As my family held nurses in the very highest esteem, perhaps I saw this as a way to please or win approval. Whatever the reason, I have no recollection of ever seriously considering any other work.

At a very young seventeen I entered the University of Cincinnati College of Nursing and Health, a setting I found scholastically demanding, and socially both stimulating and bewildering. In my third year, I fell in love and married. The 1950's notion that marriage renders a girl, if not mature, at least capable of commanding adult respect, held sway in many young lives at that time. When I became pregnant, my intention to continue school ran afoul of university policy and I left one year prior to graduation.

The next two years saw many adventures as an army wife and the birth of two beautiful sons. While the family was stationed in El Paso, Texas, I reentered nursing school at Hotel Dieu. The world was a frightening and unpredictable place in those days, however. Classes were in session for only a few weeks when the Berlin wall precipitated a dangerous crisis. I joined my husband in France, where we lived for a year.

Returning to the States and to civilian life, we moved to Dallas, looking forward to calling one place home for a long time. While the likelihood of my finishing school seemed remote, the need arose for me to contribute to the family financially. I applied for a position as undergraduate nurse at St. Paul Hospital, and, to my surprise, was assigned a position in the intensive care unit. Thus began a learning experience par excellence. In those days of few specialized units, the ICU received everyone who was severely ill. Working nights for the first five years, I became quite expert at bedside nursing in the acute care setting. For the first time in my life, I mastered a recognized and valued skill. My self-esteem soared.

It was during this period that I began to dream of returning to school. The final motivation came in the form of an unexpected challenge from a person whom I admired and respected. It was just as morning report was being completed that Sister Mary Peter, my supervisor, asked what my plans were for the future. I replied that one day I hoped to return to nursing school. Looking directly into my eyes she replied simply, "You'll never finish nursing school," then turned and went about her work. I stood stunned for several moments. Later at home, unable to sleep, I still could not forget her words. How could she doubt my intention? Did I doubt it myself? Somewhere in the processing of this encounter, it became clear that unless I began, unless I actually acted, her words would become prophetic.

Thus, in 1966, I began making inquiries, sending for transcripts and scheduling appointments—a process both time-consuming and frustrating. I shudder to recall the nursing college official at Texas Woman's University (TWU) who stated that returning to a baccalaureate program after eight years out of school was likely beyond my capability and that I should "settle" for a diploma program. Deeply discouraged, I accepted her views without question. After repeating several science courses at the local community college to eliminate single credit deficiencies, I entered and completed the program at St. Paul Hospital School of Nursing.

Passing state board exams in 1968 was a milestone. It had been a long, hard journey. Before long, however, I felt the inner rumblings of change. Constant acute care crises and working short-handed had begun to wear my enthusiasm thin. I found myself more interested in being present for many of the "problem" situations other nurses tried to avoid—people in pain or dying and families with mixed feelings about their loved ones' illnesses. Following this inclination, I entered TWU to finish the baccalaureate program and work toward a master of science in psychiatric and mental health nursing.

The last two years of school I completed while in process of a painful divorce. While hardly the ideal setting for cognitive learning, it was an effective crucible for developing empathy and humility. My boys were half-grown when I finally finished school in 1973, sixteen years after having begun.

The graduate degree opened opportunities to function as psychotherapist and counselor in various settings. It was during these years that I became aware of taking the stance I call "trying not to be a nurse," inadvertently making a statement about my view of both myself and the nursing profession. I sought to identify with psychotherapists of various backgrounds, hoping to measure up and be respected as one of them. For most of two decades, I worked in psychiatric and educational settings, always wondering when the next job might bring inspiration and meaning to my work life.

The problem, of course, was not with the work itself. Through some blend of cultural, familial, perhaps ancestral and archetypal influences, I had learned to place strict, narrow limits on the possibilities for my own life experience. From today's perspective I wonder how many other nurses, largely women, move through the years half-consciously haunted by this same disabling view.

I toyed with the thought of returning to school in clinical or phenomenonological psychology, but over time ruled out any such direction. What I really longed for was not a whole new arena of requirements and hurdles, but to feel competent and whole as who I in fact already was. The inspiration and meaning were not to be brought to me but rather awakened from within me.

It took a very personal experience to break through this impasse. In 1989 I had returned with my new husband and two stepsons to live in Kentucky. By spring of 1992, my mother lay dying of advanced breast cancer. I traveled with increasing frequency from Louisville to Cincinnati to be with her and care for her. Many of those about me there, family, physicians, and hospital staff, declined to acknowledge the obvious, that her death was close at hand. With loving support by phone from my husband, however, I cherished those final weeks with my mother. For the first time in memory I allowed myself to be completely present in the moment and fully engage the pain. This surrender became the vehicle for a beginning transformation.

In the weeks that followed, I found myself in turmoil. With both parents gone, I was in some real sense "next." When an abnormal mammogram some months later brought two weeks of cold fear before I learned I was healthy, a personal crisis ensued. Never before had I been brought face-to-face with my own mortality. Clearly, life would never be the same again. I became acutely aware that I could not bear to continue withholding so much from life. Who was I? What was I to do? Truly, if there were anything I wanted, the time was now.

As life has taught so many times before and since, the path becomes clear when I am ready to see. Following a recurring inclination to work by myself, I developed a true shoestring budget and opened a business. In designing Wellness Pathways, I hoped to offer a setting in which healing and wholeness could thrive, while rekindling some of the enduring joy I had found in nursing. To do this I drew on experience and skills as varied as therapeutic touch and bodywork, relationship-centered counseling, and development of educational programs.

Synchronistically, around this time I learned of the new American Holistic Nurses' Association Holistic Nurse Certificate Program, and rather tentatively registered for the first phase to be offered in Nashville, Tennessee. Nothing I had previously known of nursing could have prepared me for this experience. I came to the weekend largely unaware of a longstanding hunger for nurse mentors, even women mentors. Here, in this room, were three at once with whom I could relate not only with integrity but with joy! These were women with whom I could work and play, cry and laugh, dance and dream. Instantly and intuitively, I felt myself respond not to their credentials, not even to their words and actions, but to their powerful loving presence. I saw that it was possible to continue in nursing and honor myself for who I was. Truly I had found the next step and intensely creative people began to emerge from the woodwork. After decades of not knowing how to nurture female friendships, women appeared and sought to be my friend. Such welcome happenings confirmed that something was certainly right about the direction I was traveling.

Now, several years later, I have completed certification as a Holistic Nurse, a process that had brought much richness and growth. At this writing I am working with two friends, a family physician and a family therapist, in seeking to form a collaborative practice in which we meet people and address their health concerns in as complete and whole a way as possible. I have no idea what is next or where I will be a month or a year from now. What feels right for me changes, if I am willing to listen. I do know that virtually any work situation, relationship, or other life setting can be a vehicle for my work on myself.

Allowing myself to be described as a nurse healer is not something I take lightly. Healing, in my present understanding, arises naturally out of loving intention and has its source not in me, but in God. Nursing provides rich opportunity for me to be present with healing as a witness/conduit/midwife/coparticipant/concelebrant—none of which accurately or fully describes what takes place, but all of which point in some partial way to the mystery which is healing. I see that healing in nursing involves not a "doing for" so much as a "dancing with." My own life is enriched and enlivened to the extent that I allow such a reciprocal moment. I am deeply grateful for the self-healing evoked by those persons I have called patients and who have called me nurse.

In addition, I continue to learn that healing may not look like we expected it would, but takes its own form in its own time. Rather than seeking or asking for a specific outcome, we open ourselves to healing when we surrender to being loved beyond imagining, to trusting God and letting the unfolding happen as it will. I am aware of an ongoing need to recognize the limits I

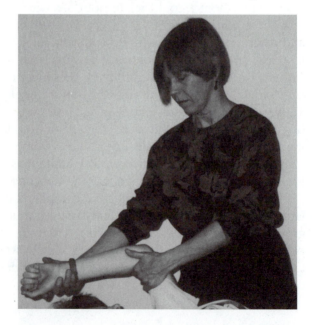

place on my life experience, reminding myself to trust intuition and grace. Often I am utterly surprised when reality manifests in a good far beyond anything I would have dreamed.

Working on ourselves, I believe, is of primary importance and extends throughout our lives. While we cannot wait until we are perfect to live our lives, it is most urgent that we actively set about seeing to our own spirit journey. We nurses so easily confuse true giving, from a full heart, with a kind of self-victimization that leaves no one the richer. I have found that when l am consistently overscheduled, fatigued, or spiritually dry, this shows up in all aspects of my life, including work settings, as an undercurrent of irritability and resentment. It is only when I have attended to my own heart and soul that there is a full, natural flowing outward toward others.

For me this has come to mean a daily practice of vipassana meditation along with the support of frequent sessions in a group setting. This practice is both the most demanding and the most transformative I have ever known. I believe it is absolutely necessary to find a spiritual practice through which to learn to listen to our own hearts and minds, to be willing to hear whatever arises and meet it with compassion. In nursing we are called upon to be present with others as they meet many of their own life lessons. I am convinced that we cannot go with another any farther than we have journeyed alone. For me to neglect my own spiritual work renders me less than helpful when called upon to be with another.

Likewise, withholding that which I can offer is to be untrue to my own light. Far too long I walked this road, avoiding a wholehearted participation in countless moments. While on the face of it this stance is craven and fearful, reframed it can as easily be seen as cold and arrogant. Being present to the healing moment requires of me that I honor who I am, what I bring, and the infinite possibilities present in participation with the other.

Equally necessary is the letting go of my assumptions, opinions, and prejudices. Not a once-and-for-all occurrence, this difficult task needs my constant attention. Healing seems to require a consistent cultivation of the open heart. When anyone, or anything is being shut out of my heart, I am to that extent closed to the movement of love which heals the whole being. Both my healing and that of the other depend on my willingness to put absolutely everything on the table, so to speak. No little pockets of sulking or resentment, no cherishing of grudges, no commerce in past hurts. Forgiveness and gratefulness, hallmarks of the open heart, precede all true healing.

Nurses, would-be healers, make room in your life for these and other influences that nourish your own wholeness—silence and aloneness, music and dance, laughter and tears, touch, passion, walks in the woods or by the sea, the presence of children and old persons, prayer and contemplation. Listen to your heart and love your body. Remember that very little is as it seems. Contrary to what we've been told, there is no real separation. What's true for you today, is true for me tomorrow. Live gratefully, walk simply, and love with great abandon. Healing and wholeness will follow.

Karilee Halo Shames
RN, PhD, HNC

*Director, Nurse Empowerment
Workshops and Services, Private
Practice, Mill Valley, California*

I was born in Miami, Florida, as
"Carole," but later changed my entire
name, thus marking the beginning of a
new era in my life, one in which I was
in charge and self-actualized. This internal
restructuring was a direct result of the chal-
lenges I faced early in my career, while providing institutionalized
nursing care, when I decided to make a difference in the world
of nursing.

It was not sufficient for me to keep my true nature quiet, to
be obedient and docile within a megacorporation. I realized that
my path was obviously elsewhere; that I needed to practice with
hands and heart from some unique perspective, one that may not
be common, perhaps not even developed by that time.

I wanted to become a nurse because I truly loved helping
people. At age thirteen, I started volunteering weekends in hospitals, fluffing pillows and holding straws, reading cards to bring
joy to people less fortunate than myself. I did this rewarding work
through my high school years, eventually being paid as a nurse's
aide. There was no doubt in my mind that I was headed for nursing school. However, with support from some of my teachers, I
was convinced to find a way to attend college and obtain a more
complete education.

Money was tight, so my fierce independent streak encouraged
me to seek out scholarships. I read countless books, and applied
for many funds. I was eventually invited to participate in a special
scholarship program through the U.S. Army. Young and naive, I
accepted it as the best opportunity available to me. I remember my
father saying "No daughter of mine will ever be in the Army," but
he was proven wrong. I stood firm in my decision, and eventually
he saw the wisdom of this plan, and offered support.

The Army was a strange place, a strong awakening for an
innocent young girl. The first two years of college were spent at

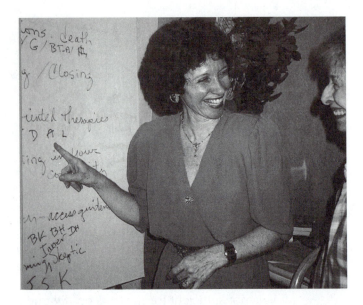

the University of Maryland, where I was treated just like thousands of other students. However, by junior year, I transferred to Walter Reed Army Medical Center in Washington, D.C., where I was to complete my final years in conjunction with the university.

The year was 1969, and the Vietnam War had deeply affected our nation. I remember first walking into a ward at the hospital, seeing forty men lined up in beds in various stages of disrepair. Everywhere I looked, there were men with arms or legs missing, with faces blown off, and tubes in every orifice. I was terrified. Our instructors had tried to prepare us, but nothing could prepare one for such a sight. My earliest Army nursing memory was of someone handing me a washcloth and telling me to "wash stumps." I suddenly realized I was not in college anymore; I was in the Army.

There were many experiences that contributed to my decision to leave before entering the final year. One of the major factors was that we had been assured we would never be sent to Vietnam, yet most of the class graduating before ours received orders to go to war. I also recall wanting to donate my body to science. I went into the office of the Judge Advocate General and pronounced my desire, which was met with laughter. Finally, he looked at me and said "You can't do that. You don't own your body. It belongs to the U.S. Army."

I was appalled, and decided to reclaim my life. After I left, I returned to the University and studied Sociology, receiving a BA cum laude within one long year. I then returned to the school of nursing and finished my senior year. Again, I was blessed to have an instructor who took me under her wing, suggesting I was talented in psychiatric nursing and should pursue an advanced degree. I was able to receive financial help, and thoroughly enjoyed my classes in individual and group psychotherapy.

However, there was always something missing for me. Inwardly, I yearned for some way of working with people that met them at their fullest; that encouraged them to make their best decisions, and to feel more at peace in health and when facing illness. I knew I could be an instrument of healing, and made efforts to develop a spiritual connection deep within myself, so that I could best inspire healing in others.

Even with an MS in Psychiatric Nursing, I felt I was somehow cheating myself, and my patients, by not inspiring something deeper. I felt constrained, unable to work freely within the confines of medical institutions. There were so many rules and violations of our sacred trust, and my being sang out for a different way. I knew there was more that could be done, and I listened to the wisdom of my heart, allowing it to guide me to more sacred ground.

The opportunity came in a surprising manner. I became ill, challenged with an autoimmune disease. I took a year off from nursing and used that time for self-healing. I studied homeopathy and spirituality and learned to use my body as a laboratory, listening to its wisdom and following its guidance. Eventually, I ended up working in a holistic center, perhaps one of the first in the nation. I knew then that I had come home.

I have continued to work holistically since that time and the rewards are immeasurable. Presently, I work in a collaborative practice with my holistic-physician husband. Working together with many of the same clients, we feel we are able to provide a very comprehensive, supportive experience. The model is empowering and enjoyable. Whereas people see him for holistic medical care, they see me for some hands-on, focused healing time. I use imagery, energy healing, counseling, and many of the tools I've gathered in the last twenty years. I feel I can take twice as long for much less cost, thus affording us more time and opportunity to explore, integrate, and release causative factors that might be more subtle and less conscious. I love what I do, and look forward to the specialness of each client and every day. I also provide healing workshops for health professionals and write books about healing.

I have had many experiences to teach me about the sacred work of the healer, but perhaps none so profound as those within my own personal life. In working with my disease, I have learned to find ease in my life. In working with my pain, I have learned how valuable my pain has been. In sharing my journey, I have made many friends, each of whom continues to teach me about the path of the healer. In working with clients, I have learned to respect their process and to help them to respect their own. In working with energy, I have allowed my intuition and my emotions to be my greatest teacher.

I have found that the greatest gift I can offer is to express myself fully, with as much love and compassion as I can muster. I am always stretching, putting myself in situations where I will learn and grow, where hopefully there is enough nourishment to sustain me through the challenges and into a deeper understanding of the miraculous interconnections of life. I am committed to traveling on an "accelerated learning" path, for I have learned to forgive myself my weaknesses, and to use my own love to transform beliefs so they serve the greatest good. Love and forgiveness have been the keys.

To those nurse healers who have yet to spread their wings and fly, I share this heartfelt message: No one else can tell you how you should do your work, or how you should live your life. Each of us is blessed with special gifts, and the world will only work its miracles when we each accept ourselves, and each other, with pure love and support. We may not always agree with each other, but we can learn to honor the unique path each of us travels as we reclaim that which is already within us—our inner healer, our highest self, and our greatest joy. I wish you tremendous fulfillment on this miraculous journey. Be sure to allow yourself to receive as much as you give, and to remember to laugh along the way, for surely it lightens our load.

Nursing is a powerful profession, and we are collectively in the process of redefining nursing for a new era. We will rise to our highest level when we individually, and collectively, acknowledge and graciously use our special talents and gifts. May the "Nurse" be with you, and may your load be light!

Marilee Tolen
RN, HNC, CHTP/I

CEO/President, Corporate
Wellness Consultants, Inc.
Cherry Hill, New Jersey

My name *Marilee* was given to me by my mother Mary Tolen (nee Haley), who somehow combined her first and maiden name to come up with mine, or so she tells me. Being a descendant of the Haley family has been about being part of a matriarchal system, different from most systems found in Irish-Scotch tradition. The matriarchal part came easy, for most of the Haley clan are/were women. I have always been proud to be what we often refer to in our family as a "Haley" woman. Even as a little girl I always had a sense of history and strong bonding among the women in our family, many of whom were in service and of vision, all of whom were very spiritual and intuitive. My senses and suspicions were confirmed when I studied the history of healing and learned that the word heal is derived from the word "hale," which means whole.

I was born in Trenton, New Jersey, and spent most of my life growing up in Cherry Hill, New Jersey. My parents offered me a great balance of practicality and creativity. Dad represented the linear, organized, and responsible structure while Mom presented the more free flowing and imaginative song and joy. There was a great blend of the masculine and feminine both housed in deep love. So, as much as I wanted to become a dancer, the more practical part of me—Dad's part—led me toward what I could count on in terms of making a living, and that was my other choice, nursing. However that practical part did not even have a voice until I knew what nursing and caretaking was like. I worked all through my high school years in a nursing home starting at the age of fourteen. I also was taking modern jazz dance classes from a teacher in New York all through high school. So my teen years were about nursing and dancing. In my junior year an interesting dimension showed itself to me when I took a class in Transcendental Meditation, received a mantra, and began an internal journey.

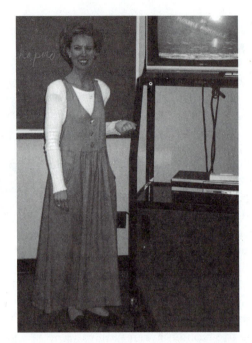

My life changed drastically when I entered Cooper Medical Center School of Nursing, a three-year diploma program. I lost my chunkiness and acne and had a heightened self-esteem (I always believed this had to do with the meditation). I became president of my class for the entire program, made great friends, and had lots of giggles and devilish water fights in the dorm. It was the mid 1970s and the disco scene was big, so after what seemed like hundreds of hours of ongoing studying we would sneak past the housemothers once a month and go out dancing at a disco. Just as I would find time to bring in the dancing, I would also find time to nourish my budding spirituality. My "spiritual" times were my meditations and listening to Seals and Crofts while watching gorgeous sunrises and sunsets over Camden, New Jersey and Philadelphia, Pennsylvania. I loved most of the classes and course work in nursing school but sometimes it was so hard I would just sit and cry wondering if I would ever get through. The specialty that I favored in school was Psychiatric Nursing, and I worked as an assistant on the psych floor the last year and a half of my training. I also won the Psychiatric Nursing award at graduation. I chose, however, to work in the Intensive Care Unit when I graduated for I wanted to have sharpened skills and more respect from the physicians.

Intensive Care was a very exciting place to work. We had a fourteen bed unit and were the designated Shock and Trauma Unit for our tri-state area, so we were very busy. It was not unusual to have two or three codes going on at the same time. I became assistant head nurse and the nursing administration was interested in grooming me for advancements, but I was clear that the administrative route was not my path. I loved ICU but developed the emotional shutdown that is sometimes necessary to cope in that environment. But I never lost my compassion. My heart still broke when I assisted in what I thought were unnecessary invasive techniques, like placing a Swan-Ganz catheter into a frail 90 year old who just wanted to die with dignity. Speaking of death, I always had a knowing and a sense of the patient's spirit/soul when they would leave their body, either while being coded or in dying. At times I would see them in witness to themselves.

After one year in ICU in 1978 I found a workshop brochure in the nurses lounge on Holistic Nursing. In the description it mentioned meditation and nutrition (I just had been reading about the benefits of juice fasting) and I knew I had to attend. It was given by a pediatric physician from Maryland who was traveling the east coast giving these workshops to nurses. The information resonated with me like no other information that I had ever received in my training. I was very excited, but that excitement turned to dismay when I realized that it was nearly impossible to apply these concepts to my nursing, for at that time the system did not have the container to hold these ideas. A few years later when I discovered the American Holistic Nurses' Association I found out that there were others who believed as I did and realized also that if I couldn't apply this philosophy in mainstream nursing I could certainly could apply this to myself. So began my personal healing journey.

As my colleagues went on for their higher degrees, I chose to study Holistic Healing, Therapeutic Touch, Foot Reflexology, Massage, Reiki, Nutrition, Edgar Cayce Remedies, and any other complementary modality that I could find. I must say that there was a great challenge here in following my heart and not in following the system. At that time there were no academic programs in these studies, so I took the "road less traveled," but now I can certainly say that it was well worth it.

I was in the first class to graduate in the AHNA Holistic Nursing Certificate Program in 1992, and received my certification as a Holistic Nurse in 1995. I also became a Certified Healing

Touch Practitioner and Instructor. I have just completed a four-year training program in Healing Science with Barbara Brennan, an atmospheric physicist whose Long Island, New York school is world renowned for teaching how to develop High Sense Perception and how to heal through the human energy field. My love and specialty is what I like to broadly term Subtle Energy Healing. I have a very busy private practice, I do a tremendous amount of teaching and have founded a corporation known as Corporate Wellness Consultants, Inc.

I would be remiss if I did not point out the element of risk that was involved for me in this journey, from not being surrounded with colleagues of like minds, and having to create and design my own work. It seems to have balanced out, however, because many of those colleagues are now worried about their jobs as nurses, and some I know are even working outside the profession. As the Northeast Regional Director for the American Holistic Nurses' Association I've been a reference point as well as a disseminator of information on holistic nursing. It's been a real joy to receive inquiries from my nursing instructors from twenty years ago requesting information on educational programs in holistic nursing!

There is a certain entrepreneurial spirit that the world of holistic nursing brings forth. I see it as creating tremendous opportunity for us to heal and empower ourselves on all levels. And as we do so the ripple effect occurs. Just like in resonant field frequency, when we heal ourselves healing occurs throughout our systems and can resonate to global proportions.

I would encourage any nurse to follow her or his heart to healership. It's embedded in our history, for even Florence Nightingale laid the groundwork in her own personal and professional philosophy.

My future work will be about assisting people to follow their longing and connecting with their purpose. I support you in this process, even and especially if it leads you on the "road less traveled." But my sense is that you'll find more nurses on the "road" as holistic nursing and modalities are increasingly requested by clients and more accepted by the conventional medical model.

Marsha Jelonek Walker
RN, MSN, RMT

Holistic Nurse Educator,
Registered Massage Therapist
Austin, Texas

My name is Marsha Ellen Jelonek Walker. I was born October 26, 1953, in Houston, Texas. My journey of becoming a nurse healer began very early in my life. My mother, aunt, and grandmother were all teachers. My mother used her teaching skills as she patiently and lovingly answered all my curious questions, and taught me about the world. I learned that all questions are important, and learning and teaching are fun. In many instances in my life my father would tell me, and demonstrate with his actions, three things that have affected my life always: (1) doing the work you love to do is more important than money, (2) you can do anything you really want to do, and (3) life is full of surprises, and to be lived by following your heart, with gusto.

My grandmother walked with the country doctor down in the "holler" to help deliver babies and care for the sick. For as long as I can remember my grandmother and parents rubbed my back at night before I went to sleep. The relaxing and healing power of touch, and the love it conveys, became part of my life very early on. I taught my girlfriends to rub backs, and we would trade at slumber parties.

I grew up in a neighborhood of boys, and I loved being the nurse in all the army games they played. When I was 14 we were asked to choose high school courses based on "what we wanted to be when we grew up." I knew immediately that I wanted to be a nurse so I could help people feel better. Nothing else seemed as important.

The summer after my first year in college I worked as a nurse's aide on the cardiac floor at Methodist Hospital in Houston. There was a man from Italy waiting to have heart surgery. His family hadn't arrived yet. He couldn't speak English and I couldn't speak Italian. I would hold his hand, and smile and wave when I passed his room. After his wife came over, she said he had told her how much I helped him. The joy I felt confirmed my plans to become a nurse. I knew then that loving people who are sick and being there for them is what they need most and what helps them heal.

After my first two years in college, I had to wait a semester before nursing school. I took a course in Buddhist philosophy and was introduced to the ideas of being conscious and aware in the moment, that we are all connected, and to the power of thought. In these classes I first contemplated that our bodies and our thoughts are energy, and what we think and feel affect our bodies and how we experience our worlds. I entered nursing school in 1975, and for my teaching project, I chose to teach a class to my peers. Drawing on my philosophy class, and my past experiences, I taught my first class in the healing power of touch and caring.

I graduated from the University of Texas School of Nursing at Austin in 1977 and began working in the hospital on a medical/surgical floor. That fall I took my first massage class and began working on friends. I had a friend with hemorrhoids who wanted to try to heal them without surgery. As a result of reading everything we could find about how to do this, I first experienced the world of herbs, vegetarianism, fasting, and holistic health. My friend healed his hemorrhoids. My acne and lifelong constipation disappeared. My world of helping people and healing had just expanded. I was very excited!

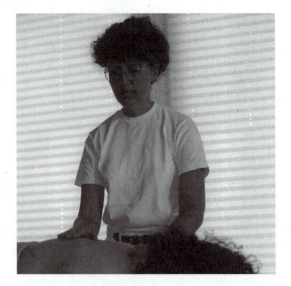

I started talking to my patients in the hospital about herbs and holistic healing. After they asked their physicians about it, I was quickly told by the physicians not to mention these things to their patients again. I started telling my head nurse about the information I had learned. She thought it was interesting, but had no place in the hospital. I was also having to spend less time with my patients. There were only two RNs, and I had to take on more of an administrative role. I discovered that what I loved about nursing was having time to talk with people, to listen to them, to rub their backs. I realized that the hospital was not for me, at this time.

In 1978, I began working for a temporary nursing service where I could more easily share what I was learning. I got a taste of many facets of hospital nursing as well as home health. The seeds of holistic healing were being planted in Austin. There were only a few of us doing massage, but my practice was growing. Massage "parlors" were about the only massage people had heard of. At first, when I said I did massage even though I said I was a nurse, people thought I worked in a parlor. Many people thought I was crazy when I talked about decreasing the amount of meat, eggs, sugar, and preservatives they ate. I realized that we are sometimes afraid of new things and from that fear, often attack others. I overcame these obstacles by continuing to tell people about the positive changes I had seen in my own body and that of clients I worked with as a result of trying holistic healing techniques. For the mutual support and shared enthusiasm, I chose to be around people who were exploring the same things I was exploring. My inner feeling continued to tell me that I was doing the right thing.

In 1978 I met Stanley Burroughs, and began to study reflexology, color therapy, and nutrition with him. That year, Dolores Krieger came to the University of Texas School of Nursing and gave a workshop on Therapeutic Touch that I attended. I was enthralled, and studied with her and Dora Kunz that summer in Washington state. I loved it! Feeling the energy field and seeing changes in myself and others showed me the next path on my healing journey. I attended the Rosalyn Bruyere Soma School of Massage in Oakland, California, and continued my training with Dolores Krieger and Stanley Burroughs. I studied breathing techniques and experienced the power of the breath as an aid to healing. That fall I began teaching massage, Therapeutic Touch, color therapy, reflexology, and holistic nutrition in several states of the U. S. and Canada.

In 1982, I began a full-time private practice doing massage, energy work, stress management consultations, and teaching in Austin, Texas. I found what I had lost in the hospital—as much time as I wanted to hear what people needed and try to help them discover how to get it. I realized I had found the way to continue being a nurse; only the setting had changed.

I started noticing the healing role in my practice and my personal life in many ways. Pain disappeared in specific areas of the client's body when I stimulated the corresponding reflex points of a client's foot. A man with emphysema was afraid he couldn't breathe; he was asleep in 20 minutes with energy work. Talking about unmet needs, a postsurgical client found the strength to make difficult changes. Herbs and energy work helped a client with a Type III Pap smear return to normal in three weeks.

In my personal life, I noticed that as my physical body began to heal, my mental and emotional life began to change also. I started noticing old ruts in my behavior patterns that kept creating unhappiness for me and those around me. I discovered that my communication skills were almost nonexistent in threatening situations. I began to learn how to express my needs and feelings, and to listen to others. As a result, miraculous changes and healing occurred in my relationships. I became aware of how long it takes to change past habits, yet how incredibly rewarding it is.

In the late 1980s I taught some Therapeutic Touch and massage workshops in the Continuing Education (CE) Department at the University of Texas (UT) School of Nursing. In 1989 I went back to school for a master's degree in Nursing. I studied psychoneuroimmunology (PNI) because I really wanted to know how thoughts affect the body. I was fascinated to learn about the link between thoughts, feelings, stress, and immune function. It was the missing piece of my puzzle. I knew I wanted to share with others what I had learned. I especially felt it was crucial information for nurses, for themselves as well as for their clients.

I rediscovered the American Holistic Nurses' Association and took two of their holistic nursing workshops and two on healing touch. I felt so thrilled to be with other nurses all talking about holistic healing in our practices. I learned many new techniques and got many new ideas.

In 1994, I helped create a holistic nursing series in the CE department at the UT School of Nursing in Austin. There are nine different workshops, of which I teach four and a half. It is a dream come true. I am able to draw on everything I have been learning and practicing for the last twenty years. In September of 1996, the UT holistic series began its third year. Several nurses have completed the entire nine month series. As many nurses in these classes begin to look at all the pieces of their lives and acquire new skills for healing, they say their whole lives change. They also say that they have rediscovered what they love about nursing—touching the hearts of those they help.

Holistic healing is not new to nursing; it is what nursing has always been. We have always known that to heal, or become whole, we must embrace all of who we are—body, mind, and spirit. Nursing, for me, is helping people identify unmet needs and discover ways to meet those needs. It is creating a space of love and safety in which a person can heal. I realized that my personal journey in becoming a nurse did not end when I graduated from school or when I left the hospital. Everything I have learned—and continue to learn—that helps myself and others to heal, is nursing.

One of the most exciting and rewarding things is to share the information I've learned. I express myself as a nurse healer in my private practice incorporating massage, energy work, reflexology, PNI information, and stress management tips. I also teach these ideas in whatever context people are interested in hearing it. Currently I'm on the faculty of the Lauterstein-Conway Massage School in Austin and, as mentioned, teach in the holistic series. I have spoken on these topics at several nursing conferences and hospitals over the last few years.

Along the way I have discovered:

- Every living thing is connected to and affected by every other living thing through the energy field, in very real, tangible ways.
- Communicating needs, feelings, and thoughts is a necessary skill for happiness and health.
- Learning to be aware in the present moment, consciously choosing our responses, is the greatest challenge and the greatest gift.
- Love is the energy that heals.

To those who would be nurse healers I would say:

- You already are one.

- Put yourself in the place of those you are with, and then act.

- No one can "heal" another. When people feel safe, they may choose to heal.

- In the uncovering and healing of what doesn't work in your own life, you learn how to help others.

- Pursue paths that are thrilling for you.

Patty Wooten
RN, BSN, CCRN

Nurse Humorist
Davis, California

Laughter brings healing energy into our body, mind, and spirit. I know, because it has given me the strength, courage, and joy to thrive during difficult periods in my life. I am a nurse humorist and a clown. For the last ten years, I have traveled throughout the United States and Europe, helping nurses, patients, and family caregivers understand and access the healing powers of humor. Comedy often arises from tragedy, and this was true in my life.

I was born in Springfield, Illinois, about a year after my father returned from World War ll. We moved to the San Francisco Bay area when I was a small baby and I have lived in California ever since. I remember daydreaming about becoming a nurse when I was in the fifth grade. I chose nursing for many reasons: a desire to help people, an interest in science, especially physiology, but perhaps the strongest reason was I wanted people to "need" me. I grew up in a severely dysfunctional family. My father was an alcoholic and my mother was a perfect codependent. My brother and I were disciplined severely and often in a manner that was physically abusive. To cope, I became an overachiever to gain my parents' approval and a "class clown" to gain attention and affection at school. Little did I know that this "clowning around" would later turn into a career.

I entered the University of California at Berkeley in 1964 to begin my journey toward a Bachelor's of Science degree in Nursing. After three years of pre-nursing study, I entered UCSF Medical Center School of Nursing. It was exciting to study nursing in a large medical center where access to scientific information was readily available. We also had clinical experience in diverse hospitals around San Francisco, and cared for patients from many different cultures and religions. But perhaps the most valuable attribute I gained from my nursing education was the awareness, skill, and motivation to become a "change agent." We were encouraged to assess the adequacy of the care environment and to create the changes necessary to improve the quality of care.

I began my career in what I believed was the most powerful setting for a nurse, the critical care unit. My first job was at Los Angeles County Hospital in the Cardiac Surgery Intensive Care Unit. This high paced, high tech environment proved to be quite a challenge for a theoretically competent but skill deficient new grad. I believed that these technical skills would make me a better nurse. I later learned that while they certainly made me more efficient and comfortable in completing my job expectations, that real nursing and true healing involved much more than manipulating tubes and administering drugs.

After about a year in the ICU, I decided to apply my nursing skills in a less technical setting. I transferred to the Health Department and became a public health nurse in Watts. I love a challenge and the chance to develop new skills. Educating and motivating indigent patients certainly was challenging, but also very enlightening. I began to understand those nursing school lectures about psycho-social-cultural factors and their impact on health care delivery. I started to believe that powerful nursing care involved so much more than drugs and equipment; it was also an interpersonal and communication skill.

It was about this time that I became pregnant, and the man I'd married in nursing school decided we should move back to the San Francisco bay area. We moved back and I began a part-time job as an ICU nurse at Alameda Hospital, a small community hospital. I was ready to take a break from challenge and drama for a while; unfortunately (or perhaps not so unfortunately) God had other plans for me. About three months after our son was born, my husband of five years decided to leave the marriage and filed for divorce. I was devastated. Dreams of a life lived "happily ever after" were destroyed. I became depressed. About six months later I moved to San Diego with my son to begin my life all over, however without my friends I was even lonelier. My life felt as though it had gone from bad to worse. I was in desperate need of a healing, for my body, mind, and spirit. It was at this low point that I heard a radio ad about clown school and I decided to enroll in the evening classes offered through San Diego State University. I received a powerful healing. I learned to laugh again; I learned to play again; I learned that I had a choice of how I perceived my reality. I could look at it directly and see only the overwhelming tragedy, or I could shift my perspective and also notice some of the delightful, amusing, and absurd moments in my life. Being a clown gave me some respite "time out" from the serious and tragic aspects of my life. As a clown, my entire focus was to create comedy and find delight in each moment, with every person. Clowns are innocent and trusting and I was able to relearn those qualities through my clown characters. Even after I took off my greasepaint, my newly awakened "inner clown" continued to help me find fun and folly in my life, and encouraged me to frolic and play. I began to heal from the emotional trauma of my divorce and childhood.

Healing is about finding balance and wholeness. We must balance work and play, rest and activity, social and alone time, introspection and productive action. We acknowledge our wholeness when we accept that our life-force encompasses body, mind, and spirit. Optimum health blends our physical, mental, and emotional energies into an integrated system. A nurse healer will support, encourage, and facilitate the blending and balancing of body, mind, and spirit.

I have chosen to express my healing energy through humor and laughter as both an educator and an entertainer. My "Jest for the Health of It!" workshops are designed to teach nurses and patients how to bring the gift of laughter to themselves and each other during stressful encounters. I consult with hospitals, clinics, and home health agencies to help them establish humor programs for patients and staff. As the president of the American Association for Therapeutic Humor, I network with other health professionals and establish guidelines and resources for practical humor applications to be applied in a variety of therapeutic modalities. As a full-time professional speaker, expressing myself verbally came easily, but learning to write was a challenge. After taking a few writing courses and finding excellent editors, I have learned the power of the pen. The *Journal of Nursing Jocularity* (a quarterly humor magazine for nurses) has provided an opportunity to write a regular column, featured in each issue. I have also edited *Heart, Humor, and Healing*, a book of inspirational quotes and funny stories. My latest book, *Compassionate Laughter—Jest for Your Health*, is a textbook and guidebook for health care professionals and family caregivers, to help them bring the healing power of

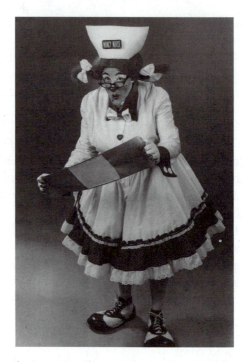

humor into their care plans. My two nurse-clown characters, "Nancy Nurse" and "Nurse Kindheart" bring the opportunity for laughter to nurses and patients. Nancy is a wild and wacky clown who helps nurses laugh at themselves and their situation. Nurse Kindheart is a gentle and whimsical clown who helps patients and their families find moments of delight and humorous perspective on their problems.

If you were to ask me for advice about what is needed to become a nurse healer I would say passion and sensitivity. You must have a strong passion for whatever medium you choose to express your healing efforts. You must believe in its power and effectiveness with your whole heart and soul. This passionate energy will stimulate you to learn, grow, and increase your skill level. Passion will be necessary to help you withstand those who doubt your work or challenge your right or ability to do it. Next, you must be sensitive—sensitive to your patient and to yourself. Let your sensitivity guide how you implement your healing modality and especially how you assess its effectiveness. Passion

Photograph of Patty Wooten as "Nancy Nurse" by Paul Herzoff

without sensitivity may cause you to overwhelm the patient with your needs and beliefs without providing opportunity for the person to discover or express inner awareness. Be sensitive to yourself and your energy levels. Sometimes in our passion to share, we may ignore internal signals that remind us of the need for rest and renewal. Always remember to maintain your sense of humor. Notice how easily your laughter bubbles up (or doesn't). Seek opportunities to laugh, either through friends, cartoons, comedians, playing with children, or simply by musing about the day and looking for humorous moments. Let me leave you with this short poem by Serene West, who expresses my beliefs so succinctly.

> Laughter is a melody,
> A concert from the heart,
> A tickling by the angels,
> Creative, living art.
> Laughter heals and comforts,
> Sometimes gentle, sometimes bold.
> Laughter is a healing dance,
> Performed within the soul.
>
> *Source: Reprinted by permission of Richard West*

Profiles

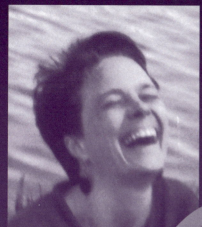

Veda L. Andrus
RN, EdD, HNC

Irene Wade Belcher
RN, MS, CNS

Dorothea Hover-Kramer
RN, EdD, CHTP/I

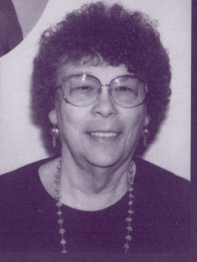

Mary J. Frost
RN, MS, CHTP/I

Ruth L. Johnson
RN, PhD

Maggie McKivergin
RN, MS

Susan Morales
RN, MSN, CHTP/I

Karilee Halo Shames
RN, PhD, HNC

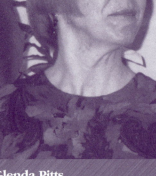

Glenda Pitts
RN, MSN, HNC

Marilee Tolen
RN, HNC, CHTP/I

Profiles

Marsha Jelonek
Walker
RN, MSN, RMT

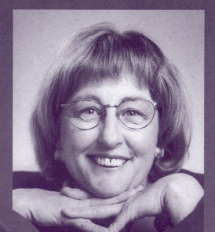

Patty Wooten
RN, BSN, CCRN

Margaret A. Burkhart
RN, PhD, CS

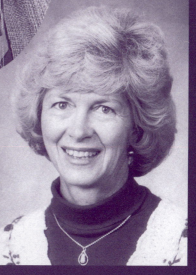

Helen Lorraine Erickson
RN, PhD, HNC, FAAN

Anne L. Day
RN, MA, PNP, CMT, CHTP/I

Merla R. Hoffman
RN, MSN, HNC,
CHTP/I

Wendy Wetzel
RN, MSN, FNP, HNC

Lynn Rew
RN, EdD, C, HNC, FAAN

Janet Quinn
RN, PhD, FAAN

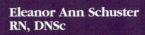
Eleanor Ann Schuster
RN, DNSc

**Donna Taliaferro
RN, PhD, CNS**

**Sharon Scandrett-
Hibdon
RN, PhD, FNP, CHTP/I**

**Melodie Olson
RN, PhD**

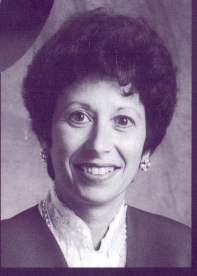

**Sandra Lutz
RN, MS, CFNP, CHTP/I**

**Joan Vitello-Cicciu
RN, MSN, CCRN, CS, FAAN**

Cathie E. Guzzetta
RN, PhD, FAAN

Jill Strawn
RN, MSN, CS

Wailua Brandman
RN, MSN, CS, NP

Rita L. Kluny
RN, BSN, CHTP/I

Rita Benor
RGN, RM, RNT, RHV, Cert Ed.
Couns. Cert, M. BAFATT

Profiles

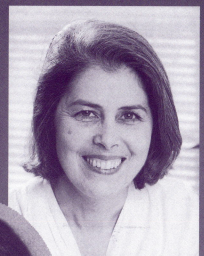

Susan B. Collins
RN, MS, FNP, HNC

Martha Fortune
RN, MS

Anneke Young
RN, BSN, CNAT

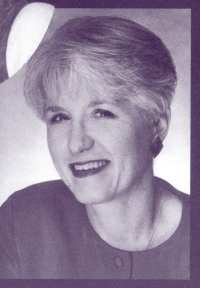

Susan Luck
RN, MA

Carol Wells-Federman
RN, MS, MEd, CS

Jean Sayre-Adams
RN, MA

Ernestina Handy
Briones
RN, PhD

Bonnie Wesorick
RN, MS

JoEllen Koerner
RN, PhD, FAAN

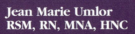

Jean Marie Umlor
RSM, RN, MNA, HNC

Chapter

4

NURSE
EDUCATORS

INTRODUCTION

How often does a student go into a classroom or a clinical practice site and think, "My instructor can never understand me, they
are only here to give information and test me." All faculty have
been in clinical practice before moving into educator roles, and
many move back and forth across the lines a number of times
during their careers. The teacher is not just a giver of facts and
tester of digested information. The teacher is frequently the guide
or the mentor into new and previously unexplored domains, who
shapes visions and opens doors to knowledge. Think of splendid
educators you have known, then move ahead to gain a glimpse
into what may make them tick.

The educators featured in this chapter are well known to
some as speakers, researchers, and authors. You may have had
the direct benefit of their teaching if you were their student or
heard them speak at a workshop or conference, or you may have
learned from their books or journal articles if you have read their
writings. If you have not done this, we suggest that if you are
stimulated by their personal stories that you look further for more
insights from them. Do a library literature review and find their
publications. Read them, then return to their portrait and reread
it. Put their cognitive contributions together with their personal
story and you will begin to discover a holistic dimension to people you may only have seen before as a teacher or author of a

publication. The educators featured here are not only teachers, but healers. Perhaps they do not represent all educators, but certainly they provide a role model for all who would be teachers.

Margaret A. Burkhardt
RN, PhD, CS,

Associate Professor, School of Nursing, Robert C. Byrd Health Sciences Center of West Virginia University, Charleston, West Virginia

Children are often asked the question "What do you want to be when you grow up?" with the sense that they will eventually choose a direction, profession, or path for their life's journey. Although we may be under the illusion that we are the ones making the choices, I have come to appreciate that, in many ways, life paths choose us. I recall hearing my sixth grade teacher describe Dr. Tom Dooley's medical missionary work in Laos, and I think I saw myself following a similar path of service to those in great need. After considering being a teacher, nun, mother, I decided by age 11 or 12 that I wanted to be a nurse. I had no family members or close friends who were health care professionals, but nursing presented itself as the path for me.

My path led to Georgetown University from 1966 to 1970. These dates are significant for several reasons. It was right after Vatican II, which, for Roman Catholics like myself, was a time of opening to the Spirit's presence in a new and exciting way.

Being in Washington, D.C., put me right in the midst of numerous protests and demonstrations calling for changes in national policy. Along with nursing courses, I learned about social justice and human rights, and questioned the status quo in many arenas. Experiences during these years contributed to a deeper appreciation of my own spirituality and its flow through all of my life and activities, and I began to more consciously ask how I was being called to respond.

My journey led me into public health nursing following graduation. Through my student experiences I discovered that health is lived in the home and community, thus, helping people to live in healthy ways is best done in this environment. I have practiced in the community since my first public health nursing job in

Connecticut, where I grew up. Other experiences along my professional path include field health nursing with the Navajo people through Indian Health Service, nurse practitioner roles within an inner city clinic in upstate New York and in a rural primary care clinic in West Virginia, and teaching nursing at the collegiate level. The journey has taken me through several academic programs culminating in bachelor and master's degrees in nursing, a master's degree in theology, and a doctoral degree in nursing, each providing opportunities to explore different facets of healing.

Many experiences have been formative in shaping my understandings of health and wholeness. From the Navajo tradition I learned that healing relates to harmony within oneself and one's surroundings, that healing requires attentiveness to spirit as well as to body and mind, and that healing and curing are not synonymous. Over the years my personal spirituality has deepened through personal and shared prayer, ritual reading, reflection, and experiences with contemplative prayer and healing prayer. The seven years that I belonged to an order of religious sisters provided opportunities for intentionally being in touch with the spiritual, and for deepening my appreciation of being apart with God/Spirit as an important part of being with others in healing ways. Through personal counseling I have come to realize the importance of receiving care and nurturing from another spiritually aware person as I attend to my own healing. Experiences such as my niece, Sheila's, diagnosis and treatment of leukemia have brought home the power of love, prayer, and presence in healing in very personal ways.

It is evident in the Christian scriptures that much of Jesus' ministry focused on healing in which he frequently used touch. This awareness led me to focus my master's research on the role of touch in healing, during which I was introduced to Dr. Dolores Krieger's early work on Therapeutic Touch. As I began to explore this and other healing modalities, the concept of healing contrasted with curing began to crystallize more clearly for me. While integrating nursing into the medical model of the advanced practice role, I found myself gravitating toward readings and workshops on healing and alternative therapies. Healing Touch, Guided Imagery, and T'ai Chi are some of the areas I have pursued along the way. It has been exciting to discover kindred spirits in the American Holistic Nurses' Association and with a few of my faculty colleagues. My thinking about the essential sameness of healing, wholeness, and holiness developed and expanded as I articulated this understanding to students, and through professional presentations and publications. My research in the area of spirituality continues to affirm that the healing path is a spiritual journey. The companionship of, and collaboration with, my husband Joe, a holistically oriented allopathic physician, and with my friend and colleague Mary Gail Nagai-Jacobson have helped me to trust the healing nature of my unfolding journey.

I never set out to be a healer. My journey to nursing was guided by a desire to be of service to others flowing from my spirituality. That the healing path has chosen me is clearer in retrospect. Others have told me that they experience healing through me and that I am a healer, so I accept that as both affirmation and caution. Since the healer is a conduit for, not the source of, healing I feel it important to be centered so as to be a clear channel, and not get ego wrapped up in acting like I am the source! What I am discovering is that healing is as much a letting go and being as it is doing. It is allowing a process to unfold, being there to guide and support much as a midwife is at a birth. Healing

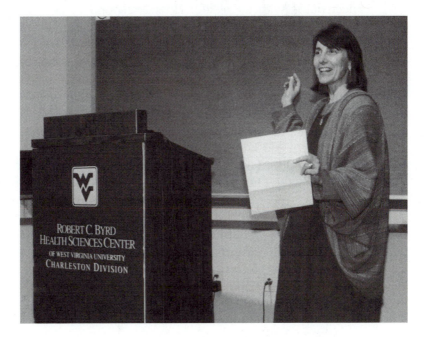

requires an ability to be with mystery. Aligning with the Light, Universal Love, God, the Christ, or however the Source of healing is imaged, is essential. Outcomes of the healing process may not manifest on the physical plane or be evident to the "healer." The intention to be with another in a loving way is the crux of healing. Particular techniques, though useful, are not essential. Nurses can be healers in the midst of performing routine care in a clinical setting if the intention to be a healing presence is clear.

I have discovered that what appeared to be two parallel paths of spirituality and healing are actually one, and that attention to spirituality, for oneself and others, is essential to healing. I express myself as a nurse healer primarily in the presence I bring to each encounter. I may incorporate modalities such as healing touch, relaxation processes, or prayer into patient encounters. I may also conduct a fairly traditional nurse practitioner visit with conscious intention to be a healing presence, acknowledging the healing force within, while listening for the patient's story and facilitating an appreciation for the body-mind-spirit connection.

Healing is about being in the world in a healing way and goes beyond patient encounters. To live in a healing way means being aware in the moment of what is, and aware of one's connectedness with all of life. How I respond to and treat other beings and the earth is important, so as part of my healing journey I consider activities such as gardening, recycling, being attentive to the environmental impact of what I buy and do, and taking time to be nurtured by the earth. Being with others in a loving way in every situation, is a goal, though not always the reality! Remember, it is the healing Source, not the healer, that is perfect! Healers need to acknowledge their own woundedness and need for healing, and nurture themselves.

The path of healing for me continues to unfold. In retrospect I see how the choices and changes are all part of a whole, not defined by job, title, or degrees. It is a Soul journey that is like a tapestry being woven of many colored threads. Many threads are constant in the pattern though the shades of some colors have changed as the tapestry unfolds. Some colors appear only for a time to enhance a section while others are recurrent. All are necessary for the design in the tapestry, which cannot be fully appreciated until the weaving is done!

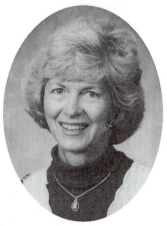

Anne L. Day
RN, MA, PNP, CMT, CHTP/I

National Instructor of Healing Touch, Journaling and Presence, Red Rock Community College Holistic Nursing Instructor, Massage, Healing Touch, and Wellness Counseling Practitioner, Founder and Owner of Healing Touch Hawaii, Golden, Colorado

I grew up in a small town in rural Minnesota, oldest of a family of five children, with grandparents and extended family close by. Ever since I can remember, I wanted to be a nurse. Memories of a Christmas present at my grandmother's house when I was 4—a doctor's kit and a nurse hat and apron that I loved! My playmates, brothers, cousins, and a young uncle (5 years older), were all male, so I was included in the backyard camping trips or imaginary spaceship adventures because they needed a nurse for emergencies. I took my position very seriously; my first aid kit got more and more sophisticated as time and maturity went on.

My young uncle, Gary, who was more like a big brother, always encouraged me to keep my ambitions and achievements high. I admired him as a role model, so when he went off to college, followed by medical school, I thought I'd become a doctor. Some of the women in his medical school classes had taken much sought-after spaces and then dropped out to have families. Gary told me not to choose medicine if I wanted to be a wife and mother, which were my other two important aspirations. That was a turning point for me. I decided to set my sights on nursing so that I could also have the family I felt was important to my fulfillment. In retrospect, I know I could have done it all, but I am forever thankful for that important decision that directed me back to nursing. I know my path has been perfect, and I couldn't be happier with my life work as a nurse healer.

In my second year at the University of Minnesota School of Nursing, I had an experience that almost changed the tide again. We had just started clinical and I had a patient with gangrenous feet. I had to leave the room and almost fainted. As I sat in the hallway, head down and green around the "gills," an insensitive intern taunted me with "You'll never make it as a nurse!" That cruel statement shook me deeply and for several months I seriously looked at changing majors to teaching. My wise nursing instructors saw my true potential and love for the field and encouraged me to stay. Two years later, I graduated with honors and was excited to enter hospital nursing as a professional baccalaureate nurse!

My first job was in obstetrics in a Lutheran hospital in St. Paul, Minnesota. I learned the ropes quickly and in six months was able to handle charge nurse positions in labor and delivery, nursery, and postpartum. I especially loved the excitement of working labor and delivery and witnessing the miracle of birth. Even more awesome was the experience of delivering a few babies in the middle of the night for doctors who didn't make it there on time!

When I was married a year and a half later, I decided to try a new area of nursing. I took a job as a public health nurse for Anoka County just north of the Twin Cities. I found I loved this area of nursing also, especially the opportunity to teach families as I visited them in their homes. My love for obstetrics and the deep desire to empower the young unwed mothers I visited inspired me to develop prenatal classes for unwed mothers. I enlisted the help of the county Social Services in the same office and in 1970 a social worker and I began a pilot project in which we offered six weeks of two-hour classes to unwed mothers. As far as I know, it was the first program of its kind in the country. Children's Magazine published an article on our classes in April 1971.

A part of me knew that teaching and speaking were special gifts for me. My early achievements in a high school speech class with an outstanding drama teacher laid the foundations. But inside of me was the passion for sharing what I loved with others. I found early on that if I truly loved what I was teaching, something greater inside me took over and flowed through, creating a pathway with others that could only be described as a heart-connection.

The desire to share more with others led me back to school a year later, after my first child was born. I was intensely interested in parenting, my new life task, so I became a Pediatric Nurse Practitioner to expand my knowledge and expertise in that area. Again, I found I could be authentic in teaching parents because I was teaching from the heart and from my own life experience, both in being a new parent and in the experience of being the oldest of five children.

Again, I was led back to teaching classes for new parents as I worked with two family practice medical clinics and then the Child Bearing, Child Rearing Center at the University of Minnesota. This innovative new program combined the expertise of nurse-midwives and pediatric nurse practitioners to provide primary care to families with physician backup. Our program was on the leading edge of health care in 1974–75. I loved being with innovative leaders, cutting new trails in health care delivery.

We moved to Denver in 1977. I continued as a PNP—teaching as a clinical preceptor for the CU nursing school's extension program to teach PNPs and working in clinic for TriCounty Health Department doing well-baby and minor illness care.

By 1982 I was in my "mid-life" crisis in nursing. I was tired of seeing parents who expected me to fix their children with the magic pill, unwilling to change the ways they were used to doing things for better health. My two closest friends were going to real estate school. Why not join them? My people skills could certainly make more money selling houses. But no, something inside reminded me of a vision strongly present, although still unclear. It has something to do with teaching and healing.

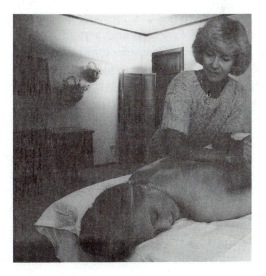

Photograph courtesy of David R. Jennings

In 1984, I took a class called Healing Touch taught by the Gotach Foundation that offered continuing education units for nurses. It got my attention! This was a true critical point in time for my unfolding destiny as a nurse-healer. That class opened up a whole new avenue of nursing for me. It stimulated my commitment to begin a master's degree in Health and Wellness. It also led me to Janet Mentgen and her early Healing Touch classes in Denver. By 1987, I was a trained local instructor, and I knew that I had truly found my passion.

Another landmark year for me was 1988. I attended my first national American Holistic Nurses' Association conference and felt that I had really come home to the heart of nursing. It was a resonance so deep and strong, I knew this group would be "family" forever. As I listened to the speakers, something deep inside was saying "Yes! Yes! Yes!"

I also heard the guidance to go beyond the classes and "Get in and swim!" with my budding knowledge as a nurse healer. With a business partner, I bought a small massage practice and was given the vision of a multidisciplinary healing center, with many different practitioners coming together to support each other and offer healing to the community. As I stepped forward in a huge leap of faith, the vision began to manifest. I was inspired with a new name—Whole Body Health Center, and a new logo, sketched on a piece of scratch paper and finalized by an artist. Being a co-owner of a growing holistic center was a great opportunity to grow, learn, and actualize the holistic knowledge and skills I had absorbed through my master's degree in Health and Wellness, that I completed in 1990. Two ancillary pieces of my training as a healer included becoming a certified massage therapist and a certified instructor in journaling as a therapeutic tool.

One of the most important things that I learned in my seven years as a business co-owner is that to be successful in a holistic business you must have a vision and you must also be grounded in good left-brained business and management skills. It is an important integration that creates a delicate balance I would call pragmatic visioning. It combines the "big picture" with the ability to deal with the day-to-day nitty-gritty details and the bottom line. All of this must be tied to the unquestionable premise of love as the foundation of all healing and therefore the core of how any holistic practice must be run. It means we must give up the illusion of lack and realize we are all here to help each other.

When Healing Touch became a national program, I began to teach around the country. It was exciting to see how Healing Touch opened people's hearts to what healing was all about. Healing Touch was changing people's lives and I was honored to be a catalyst in that process.

At the same time, I began to teach Holistic Nursing in our local community college, where the faculty decided to offer a certificate program in Holistic Nursing. In this holistic health program, I continue to be delighted to see nurses and others learn how to "wake up" to their potential and to what the essence of healing really means. I've seen nurses who feel totally burned out in nursing actually light up as they connect with the principles of holism and the many possibilities that holistic nursing holds for them. I love teaching the three levels of Holistic Nursing and seeing the commitment and maturity that develops by the time the students present their final projects in Level III. It is fulfilling to offer these openings of inner vision to others, and I experience opening and healing each time I teach it.

I believe that I have a special gift for teaching. As I teach what I know and love, I feel a wonderful energy flow through me, which creates an energy for healing as well as learning. I believe that our ultimate purpose is healing ourselves and claiming our Sacred-Selves, and when I am teaching, I feel that part of me truly radiating. Presently, I teach Journaling as a Therapeutic Tool, Journaling the Spiritual Journey, Journaling the Healing Journey, Healing Presence, Wellness Counseling, Massage Therapy and Healing Touch, along with the Holistic Nursing and the national Healing Touch classes.

I express myself as a nurse healer through a wonderful dance I do with my work: It requires the flow between hands-on individual healing sessions and group teaching or speaking. I believe that to be a great teacher, you must also be practicing what you are teaching. Therefore, I am thankful for the many Healing Touch and massage clients who faithfully fill my schedule when I'm home in the office. For me, intention is the most important element in healing—the intention to work at the highest level of love vibration that you have achieved within yourself.

Therefore a commitment to personal spiritual growth is essential for any healer. The vibration of unconditional love brings healers to a place where they can begin to resonate with that powerful energy of healing love within themselves that helps them reconnect with the divine essence of who they really are that may have been forgotten. Healers establish a presence that surrounds them with a radiant vibration which communicates that the healers are also love and have the power within to release fear and heal themselves. This is true empowerment: Helping others to move past the illusion that holds them in a space of pain and disease. As healers, I believe we are called to dance the dance, allowing the rhythm and flow of the energy to guide the healing process. We must commit to daily attunement to love and to consciously living, choosing to be heartfully responsible to ourselves and the many partners who join us in this dance.

Helen Lorraine Erickson
RN, PhD, HNC, FAAN

Professor, School of Nursing, The University of Texas at Austin, Austin, Texas

I grew up in a small, midwestern community with a strong work ethic background. As the oldest daughter and one of four children in a lower-middle income family, I learned early in life that I had familial responsibilities as well as responsibility for myself. My father, a loving, intelligent, and hard-working man with German ancestry, illustrated the importance of being committed to the integrity of the work rather than the salary. He often used his sense of humor to help himself cope with life events. My mother, a dedicated soul-mate for my father, illustrated the importance of maintaining a family unit, consistency and continuity in the family, and family values and pride. I remember her telling me, "Remember that you are no better than anyone else, but also remember that you are just as good as everyone else." My mother's sister, a nurse, was also a major player in my development. She was selfless, loving, compassionate, and intelligent.

When I was about 4 1/2 years old, I had been disciplined. As a result, I was very angry—I *knew* that the discipline was not fair! I decided that when I grew up, I would always be fair! The only person I knew who was always fair was my aunt. Since she was a nurse, that meant that I too would be a nurse! Of course I look back on the event and couple it with my mother's version, which is that I was extremely persistent in my views and know very well that the discipline was not only fair, but helped build character needed for the rest of life. Although this was clearly an important event in my life, I didn't make the conscious, cognitive decision to go to nursing school until I was a freshman in high school. My advisor asked me what I wanted to do after I graduated, and offered me three choices: continue to work in my current job as a checkout clerk in a food store, become a teacher, or become a nurse. I knew then that I would be a nurse and planned accordingly the rest of my high school years.

Throughout my life I have enjoyed people of all ages. I have worked for pay since I was 10 years of age; each job involved direct interactions with people. I enjoyed being able to help people in need, interact with people who sought a relationship with me, and most important, I have always known that I was meant to help people. I merely operationalized this when I chose nursing as my life work. I view nursing as the nurturing and facilitating of people so that they can maximize their well-being. This means living a full, quality life even when one might be taking his or her last breath. I wanted to be a nurse so that I could help others in this way.

I was educated as a diploma nurse in the 1950s. This was a wonderful experience. I learned about my own strengths, and the wonderful reward of being with others when they are in need and vulnerable. I also learned that nursing is unique and that nurses deal with the person first and the equipment second. After graduation I worked in nearly every type of health care setting, in a variety of places, and learned about who I was as a nurse and person. During the early 1970s a friend (and later colleague), Mary Ann Swain, encouraged me to return to school to label and articulate what I was doing. Mary Ann would often ask about my practice and listen to my stories about the people that I cared for—how they would come to my house, or call me, or state that they had "waited until I got back on duty" to tell me what was "really" the problem. She argued that my understandings needed to be shared with others. I explained to her that others did not want to hear about my understandings! Nevertheless, after a particularly difficult experience with a group of residents, I decided that maybe I did need to go to school so I could communicate better why it was important to be concerned with human needs, to care about the spirit of the person, and to explain why people sometimes lost the will to live, gave up, and died. This decision sent me back to school to earn a BSN. Although I had earned 30 college credits in the 1950s, it was now the 1970s; the credits were not recognized, so I started over. Upon completion of my BSN it was clear that I needed to continue. Convinced that persons are holistic, I designed a combined

Psychiatric-Mental Health and Medical-Surgical master's degree. I owe thanks to Jean Wood and Maxine Loomis for their willingness to permit this aberration to the preplanned programs at The University of Michigan School of Nursing.

There are three interwoven threads that have created the tapestry of who I am as a nurse and person. I became aware of the first when I was a student nurse in Children's Hospital in Detroit. One night about midway through our rotation I had a dream that was very clear. In the dream Christ walked through a door and said, "You have a job to do, go do it." The dream was so profound that it partially woke me from my sleep. I remember getting up, wandering down a hall and going into another building (which I later learned was the medical quarters—we were prohibited from going there). I found myself in a room with many books; as though I were in a trance, I pulled a book off a shelf and opened it. The picture in the book was the same as the dream. The caption of the picture was "Let your light so shine"; the text referred to a scripture in the Bible, Matthew's 5:11. I had no idea what it meant, and marked it up as "walking in my sleep." One year later I met my future father and mother-in-law. They were attending one of the first American Society for Clinical Hypnosis conferences. During that weekend I became aware of the importance of mind-body relations and my potential as a facilitator of healthy responses. Two years later I gave birth to my first child; within the next seven years we had three others. During these early formative years I often thought about each of these experiences. Being a part of the birth, growth, and development of a wonderful little human being is the most magical, awe inspiring experience possible. My work was to help my children grow to be responsible, caring human beings and also know that as they grew they would need my influence less and less was sobering. I gained great comfort from knowing that the values I might instill could ripple out and help others if I facilitated them to be uniquely individual, to be true to themselves, and to be spiritually healthy. I was also very aware that these people, my children, were not "mine," but were instead a gift sent to me to enrich my life, to help me learn and to help me grow spiritually.

Throughout the years these three factors—my early life experience with a message of sorts, an introduction to alternate ways to think about the nature of health and well-being, and the influence of my beloved children and husband—have influenced how I think, how I act, what I value, and who I am. They have helped me set priorities and to articulate what I believe in.

During the late 1960s I became consciously aware of the number of patients who seemed to be more comfortable, who seemed to live better or die more peacefully after our interactions. At first I disowned any role in these observed responses; I wasn't ready to fight the battles that seemed necessary if I claimed that our role as nurses was to heal, not help physicians cure. Finally, however, it was impossible to deny even to myself that what was happening was not just by serendipity, but was an outcome of enactment of values and beliefs. Finally, as I indicated earlier, I reached a point where I had to decide which way to go, so I chose to return to school to find ways to label and articulate what I knew in the deepest part of my being was what I was about. I needed to find a way to help nurses heal so they could help others heal. I also needed to find a way to help nurses understand that our role is to help people grow, to love, to laugh, and to heal. This is who I am.

While some might think that going back to school was difficult, that was simply hard work. I think the major obstacles were to learn how to not personalize anger or hostility that was occasionally projected when colleagues felt left out. As an example, I worked as a part-time nurse for a number of years while my children were growing. Although I enjoyed my multiple activities with my children, I also thoroughly enjoyed my relationship with my colleagues—I was not just someone else's mother or wife, I was a professional with my own identity too. Therefore, I would look forward to the greetings and comments that my colleagues and I exchanged as I reported for duty. So one evening when I arrived for work and none of the staff would speak to me, my first thought was that I had done something wrong— maybe I had forgotten to come to work when I was supposed to. When I checked, that wasn't the case. For the next few hours I was very confused—what had I done? Then I happened to notice a letter that had been sent to the hospital personnel from a patient that I had cared for a few weeks before. He stated that he wanted to comment on the wonderful care he'd received and to mention two nurses in particular; I was one of them. When I saw the letter I knew immediately that it was somehow related to the way my colleagues were reacting to me that evening. So, I asked one of the other nurses and she said yes, they were angry that I had been mentioned—after all, I only worked part-time and I always got the "good letters." I was crushed, I always tried to be very quiet and non-obtrusive about any letters or recognition that I received. In fact, I rarely told anyone but my husband when patients would visit me at my home, call, or send notes or gifts. Nevertheless, my friends were angry with me because I had provided good care and was recognized for it. I nearly left nursing over that experience. However, after considerable soul searching and discussions with my husband, I reframed the experience. I remember my husband telling me that it was important that I continue as a nurse so that others could learn from me. That was a remarkable thought! At the time it seemed that this was the last thing my colleagues would ever want. But, I did remember that I had a responsibility—a role—and although I wasn't sure about what it was or how it would evolve, I knew that I was a nurse to help others, not to get my own needs met from my colleagues. I have had numerous other experiences where people who matter to me misinterpret my intent. I try not to personalize, to introspect and assess my own motives, and to remember that we are all humans, are all motivated by our own needs, and that in the most part, people do not intend to hurt or discount.

When I can transcend difficult experiences, important learnings occur. Spiritual well-being is the essence of happiness; for spiritual well-being to exist, healing has to occur. When people experience loss, they often need help recovering.

I teach, practice, and try to live a simple, decent, loving life. I work hard to understand and respect others, to value their uniqueness, to enjoy their being, and to accept and love them as they are. I also work hard to enjoy myself, to find ways to nurture my own growth, and to be connected to people and ideas that nurture me and help me feel fulfilled.

My message to others is to believe in yourself and be true to your own beliefs. Prioritize your life roles; be clear about what is important in your life. If you stay true to yourself and your beliefs, even the most difficult of circumstances can become meaningful experiences. Value others, look for their strengths, promote and reinforce their worthiness, and remember that all humans have an inherent need for respect and dignity.

Consider what you would like to be able to remember when you are 80, how you would like to live your life at that age—what will be important then must be attended to now.

Merla R. Hoffman
RN, MSN, HNC, CHTP/I

Holistic Nursing Consultant and Educator, Colorado Springs, Colorado

One of the discussions I remember in my study of growth and development in nursing school had to do with nature vs. nurture and which of these had more influence on a person's talents, personality, or choice of career. I imagine I found this discussion particularly interesting since I was adopted at birth and often wondered about what characteristics I inherited and which ones I learned. As far as the profession I have chosen, it looks as if I received a double dose, or maybe even a triple dose, of nursing.

I was born at Mercy Hospital in Denver, Colorado. My birth mother was a nurse. I was adopted at seven days of age by Helen and Merle Howk of Bird City, Kansas. Helen Howk is a nurse. Helen's only brother was a physician, and one of her sisters is also a nurse.

I grew up in a small wheat farming community and, for most of my youth, there was no physician who practiced in our town. Many traveled 21 miles to Benkelman, Nebraska, to "doctor with" my uncle who had his practice there. Before my birth, Mother kept an office in Bird City, and her brother came once a week to see patients. During my childhood, Mother often gave injections, checked blood pressures, and always went when the phone rang and someone had a sick child who was having a seizure, or there had been an accident. I came home from school one day to find a piece of partially hung wallpaper dangling from the wall and Mother nowhere to be found. There had been an automobile accident involving two teenage girls, and Mother had been called to come. She accompanied the girls in the ambulance to the hospital in Benkelman and then flew on to Denver with the girls in a private plane owned by a local farmer. She then stayed at one of the Denver hospitals and provided nursing care for them for a few days. She returned home to finish hanging the wallpaper a week later.

Early on, I was immersed in nursing and caring. I saw a nurse functioning independently, working closely with a supervising physician—today what we view as the nurse practitioner role. I also observed how much my mother, my uncle, and my aunt genuinely cared about their patients and their families. Even a trip to the grocery store was an opportunity for Mother to listen to people's concerns about their health; she often listened to questions and provided health education while standing in the checkout line. I learned that nursing is a way of life, not something you only do at certain times and places, and that when you care for one person, you are really caring for an entire family, usually the extended family. There was another factor that influenced my choice of nursing as a career. My father suffered with bipolar disease, and in those days before Lithium, we had many ups and downs in our family. However, through all the ups and downs, I seemed to have the ability to meet Daddy wherever he was in his cycle and to simply "be" with him. He taught me early on the power of unconditional love. He loved me unconditionally from the moment he first held me as an infant; and I soon learned that kind of love could overcome anything. Modern psychiatry and psychotropic drugs helped to keep him stable and functioning in his community, and

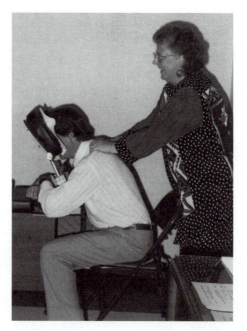

unconditional love helped him to experience joy and a level of healing. I wanted to learn more about how I could be of help to him and to others who suffered from mental illness.

The stage was set. In those days, the two primary career pathways for women were teaching and nursing. "Well," I said, "I definitely don't want to be a teacher!" That was a statement that would come back to haunt me the first day in Fundamentals of Nursing. Our instructor began class by telling us, "The nurse is a teacher every day." I almost bolted from the classroom! I wasn't there to learn to teach; I was there to learn how to facilitate the healing of people. What I soon discovered was that I loved teaching. I loved teaching my patients about their bodies, their diseases, and how to take care of their health, and I realized my Fundamentals of Nursing instructor had been "right on." A healer teaches, and the teacher heals.

After graduating from the University of Colorado with a BSN, I returned to my roots. I took a position in the 28-bed community hospital in Benkelman where my uncle had built the first hospital in the community. My aunt was the Director of Nursing. I gained a great deal of valuable experience in the year I worked there. I also observed, once again, the importance of caring, touch, therapeutic presence, and unconditional love. When my aunt went to nursing school, antibiotics were just becoming available. In the early days of her career, she often had nothing more to offer her patients than her touch and her presence, and I had seen her use both of them many times as I was growing up. My aunt often worked the shift after mine, and we always knew when she had arrived because of her quick step in the hall. I was with a patient who was feeling very ill one evening, when we heard my aunt's step in the hall. The patient's face relaxed; he sighed and smiled. "Bernie's here," he said. "I hear her step in the hall, and I feel better." Now that's presence! She never entered a patient's room without fluffing their pillow, wiping their brow, or patting their hand. When she was there, the patient was sure he was the only person she had to care for, and she had all the time needed to help him.

During the year I worked in Benkelman, I met my husband and was married. My husband was a graduate student in Boulder, and my parents suggested that if I wanted to go to graduate school, now was the time. Once again I attended the University of Colorado, earning an MSN in Maternal-Child Nursing with my focus being obstetrics and education. I taught Maternity Nursing at the University of Northern Colorado and Northern Arizona University, and loved every minute of it. During my tenure at the University of Northern Colorado, my students did their clinical at Mercy Hospital in Denver, on the unit where I was born—another return to my roots. My husband then accepted a faculty position at the University of California, Berkeley, and I began working on call in labor and delivery at Alta Bates Hospital. There were students from two different nursing schools doing clinicals on our unit, so I thought I had the best of both worlds. I had patients of my own to care for, and I had an opportunity to interact with students. It has always been important to me to provide those preparing to be nurses with care and support on their journey. They are the future nurse healers.

While I was working at Alta Bates, we decided to begin our family. I worked up until the time when physicians began pushing my labor patients to the delivery room for me because they were concerned I would go into labor. When our daughter was 9 months old, we moved to Colorado Springs and, at that point, I made the choice to be a stay-at-home mom. I began saying to people, "I used to be a nurse." However, my husband gently reminded me of what I knew deep in my heart. I would carry out some activity and he would say, "There's the nursing process in action again."

Once again, I returned to my roots: those behaviors that were so much a part of my experience growing up, and in my early nursing career—caring, therapeutic presence, touch, education, and most importantly, unconditional love. I decided to reactivate my nursing license which I had placed on inactive status. Much to my delight, I found continuing education classes for nurses on Creative Visualization, Massage, and Therapeutic Touch. I learned of an organization called the American Holistic Nurses' Association. I came home!

For several years now, some therapists in the community have called me to act as their sounding board when they have had a particularly difficult client. My husband has called me the therapist's therapist; now, he calls me the nurse's nurse. I have a private Holistic Nursing Consultation and Education practice in which I help clients with stress management, wellness counseling, and energy balancing. Many of my clients are other nurses who seek me out formally and informally for assistance and education regarding their health, and to listen to their stories. I feel very strongly that for nurses to provide excellent care for their patients and clients, they must first provide excellent care for themselves, and that is a large focus of my healing practice. I organized a local network of the AHNA in Colorado Springs, and I accept every invitation I receive to speak to groups, particularly groups of nurses, about holism and complementary healing practices and modalities. I teach Healing Touch classes in my community and am active in mentoring students in that program. I am actively involved in AHNA at the national level, serving as a member of the Leadership Council. I find my life is very full and very rewarding. Being a nurse healer is a part of who I am every minute of every day, and I am committed to continuing my efforts to facilitate and educate nurses and others regarding what I consider to be the essence of healing—caring, therapeutic presence, touch, and unconditional love.

Melodie Olson
RN, PhD

*Associate Professor, College of Nursing,
Medical University of South Carolina,
Charleston, South Carolina*

My great-aunt Margaret was a nurse. She told me about the uproar that surrounded the issue of whether or not nurses should be allowed to take blood pressures. It had been a physician's task, but nurses spent more time with the patients than the doctors did. They could get the information more quickly, and more often. On the other hand, what would the numbers mean to nurses? What would they do with the information? Now, thirty years after she told me the story, I am a member of the State Board of Nursing. Each month we get questions that begin "Is it within the role and scope of function of the Registered Nurse to . . . ?" do some task. The pattern of dynamic tension between professions that work together to share the art of healing is still repeating itself.

Patterns have always been evident in life, as we seem to revisit experiences, people and stories time after time with new understanding and growth. Mr. Bowwer (whom I wrote about in *Healing the Dying*), spent eight months dying, and teaching me what it was like to die as I cared for him in those months. I have seen his lessons with others as a part of being a nurse healer. Making the patterns clear to others is a part of being a teacher. But for the most part, his lessons touched me when I lost people close to me, my mom, brother, grandparents, aunts and uncles, dad. It was important for me to know what it was like to die.

After a few years of staff nursing, I became a teacher. I lived in Papua-New Guinea for five years, teaching nursing in a mission school. I learned one pattern there from a new graduate nurse. The new graduate said to his friend, "I am going to fly to your island every weekend that I am off duty, to see you." One teacher pointed out to him that it would consume all his pay. With no hesitation or guile, he said, "But friends are more important than money." It was his pattern to live in a way that celebrated people, and he was fully present when he was with them, friends or patients. That attitude is not limited by the country one lives in, but is sometimes easier to see somewhere other than home.

Repetition is not the same thing as repeating patterns. In my early years as a teacher in a graduate Adult Health nursing program, I focused on teaching as my major responsibility, and class content was substantially the same for several years. Yet each group of students created a different energy, enthusiasm, understanding, and growth of wisdom in those classes. Discussions of spirituality usually included content on the concept of transcendence (moving beyond self to a connection with something). Some groups merely reported on the research in the area, and suggested that it is good because of measurable outcomes. Others created a means of achieving transcendence in the class itself, and a new understanding emerged. Repetition of the topic, even when the class readings and format were the same, did not achieve the living pattern of transcendence. A teacher only creates the environment in which growth and knowledge can occur. Those present develop the new understandings.

Healing is not something any of us does to another. It occurs within an individual. But we, as nurses, do create an environment which encourages that healing, whether it is in school, a hospital, a clinic, or the community. With Therapeutic Touch (TT), the idea of repatterning the human energy field made sense to me. I had practiced TT with patients since I went to Pumpkin Hollow Farm, and learned from Dolores Krieger and everyone who was present there how to begin. It was one method of creating a healing climate which required being fully present with an individual, clearly focusing on helping that person. It also challenged me to spend more time developing my own way of centering. Many of my friends were learning meditation from a variety of ancient traditions. While I value many old and established techniques of meditation, I find my identity in the Christian faith. I started investigating some of the early traditional Christian meditation techniques, especially contemplative prayer. I read varied works: Hildegard von Bingen, Thomas Moore, Dietrich Bonhoeffer, Teilhard de Chardin, and C.S. Lewis. But not until I created my own meditations from works like the twenty-third Psalm, and learned to experience a silent retreat at Christian retreat centers, did I begin to experience the centering in God necessary for me to practice centering with the client. So that's what I do.

I became a researcher a few years ago to begin to extend my knowledge (not experience) of healing. That meant using good science to look at the outcomes believed to be related to various healing modalities. Colleagues at a large medical university helped design appropriate research methods to begin finding out what outcomes can be expected from Therapeutic Touch. This assumes there are one or more standard outcomes to a healing technique. By using the scientific method, one agrees to such an assumption. After several small pilot studies, we were fortunate to receive a grant to study TT and anxiety from the Office of Alternative Medicine at the NIH. The study tested the anti-anxiety effects of TT using immunologic outcomes. The premise was that stress impairs immune function. Therefore, relieving stress should improve immune function which has been compromised by stress. Our results were mixed, but there were some significant effects. We continue to study, not to prove that TT works, but to determine how to measure its effects, who benefits most, and other quantitative questions. Proof of its efficacy is determined by each client in his/her own life. The nature of TT is to support the healing environment, creating the internal peace so that healing can occur. Qualitative studies may capture that spirit in a more complete way than the quantitative approach.

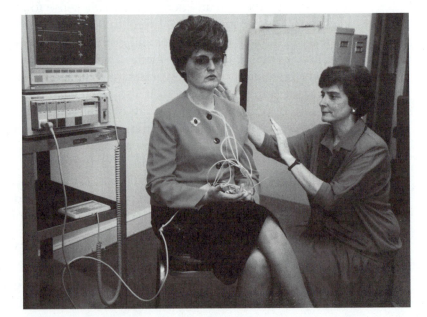

The interesting thing about researching in the area of healing, especially something like TT, is that the dynamic tension evident in life between professions and between individuals is still there, but in a different way. Scientists often question whether healing can be investigated using scientific methods. Some questions are not answerable by science. They are matters of faith. The practitioners sometimes believe that science is too limited to ask the right questions. One example would be the investigation of the Native American sweat lodge ceremony to determine if it is efficacious. A strict scientific approach would require breaking the ceremony into its component parts and analyzing each part. Yet there are no parts. What would you leave out, or what part would you study on its own? In the picture, we have a client connected by electrodes to a monitor. Does the act of doing that make the environment less conducive to healing? Would the measurement change the outcomes? Practitioners who want to be reimbursed for their work are required by the economy of our health care system to show an effect that is useful to society. So scientists think the healers use faith, and the healers think the scientists need to change their methods to get to the truth.

In my practice, we simply continue to do TT for those who would like to share the experience, teach it to those who want to learn, and look for ways to determine if there are consistent outcomes that are measurable. I think both the healers and the scientists are right. Methods of the scientist should be used where they are useful, and used well. The patterns of healing that are uncovered will help us all learn to be better healers.

Janet Quinn
RN, PhD, FAAN

*Associate Professor and Senior Scholar,
Center for Human Caring, School of
Nursing, University of Colorado Health
Science Center, Denver, Colorado*

From the time that I was five years old I wanted
to be a nurse. I did all the usual "playing nurse"
things, and then some. This included pleading for
a microscope at about age eleven or so, and subse-
quently sequestering myself in my "laboratory" discovering how things were made. True to my first-born character, when
I was in the fifth grade I wrote away to the local nursing school
to ask them what I had to study in high school to get into their
program. I don't remember the response, but I can only imagine
the faces of the admissions' folks! My mom and dad always
encouraged my pursuits, and in this case, trying to help me see
that I could do whatever I wanted with my life, suggested that I
consider becoming a doctor. I didn't want to hear of it, certain that
I wanted to be with the patients—touching, holding, soothing, and
healing, rather than in and out, which was my perception of doc-
toring. When I was hospitalized one summer for pneumonia this
observation was confirmed.

In my senior year of high school my debate partner and I won
the National Catholic Forensic League championship. I received a
list of very prestigious universities where I could go on full debate
scholarship and proceed on to law school, but my decision to
become a nurse remained firm. I began working as a nurse's aide
at the local hospital where I had previously volunteered as a "candy
striper" and went off to Hunter College-Bellevue School of Nursing.
Sometimes I think that I was the best nurse I've ever been in those
days. I was "only" a nurse's aide; I did the baths, the "vitals," the
backrubs, and the hand holding. I reassured family and spent time
visiting with them when they came. I read to patients, and I can still
remember leaving a room of four with everyone clean, refreshed,
and smiling, having been touched a lot, having laughed a lot, talked
a lot, and been cared for a lot. I loved it.

When I graduated I went to work in a busy emergency department in California and later moved to ICU/CCU. After several years of instantaneous assessment, diagnosing rhythm strips, and managing monitoring devices, I began feeling like, somehow, I had lost my direction. Was this all there was to nursing? Is this what I had aspired to since I was five years old? After teaching in a diploma program for a year, I went to graduate school at New York University.

Meeting and learning from Martha Rogers, a leading nurse theorist, was an experience—sometimes fun, sometimes challenging, sometimes painful, but never boring. My mind was completely blown as I considered ideas I had never imagined and learned a new "nonparticulate" language. Still, my disillusionment with nursing continued to grow. I was considering a doctoral program in clinical psychology when a strange thing happened. I took an elective with Dolores Krieger called "Frontiers of Nursing" in which she taught Therapeutic Touch (TT). Slowly as the semester progressed and I had actual experiences of TT and what it could do, I had a complete change of heart and mind from skeptic to committed learner.

Very shortly after I graduated, my mother was diagnosed with terminal colon cancer. I moved to California to take care of her and used lots of TT. It made a huge difference, for her and for me, and so following her death I decided to return to NYU to complete my doctoral studies in nursing. My goal was to help carry on the pioneering work of Dolores Krieger—to help Therapeutic Touch move fully into the mainstream of nursing practice, so that every patient in every hospital could access it. I had finally rediscovered nursing as healing, and had fallen in love again with what it is that we do.

I have been involved in this work for twenty-two years. Since completing my doctoral research on TT I've done several other studies, published extensively, and most recently completed a set of videotapes with the National League for Nursing. The tapes are being used to teach TT all over the world, by schools of nursing and hospitals, and now by individual health care professionals and family members. My goal, to do what I could (not all that needs to be done) to help nurses recover their healing role through the use of TT, has been met, although not without continuing difficulty.

In initial scuffles with TT opponents here in Colorado, I responded with the sense of a righteous warrior—I raised my sword and accepted the challenge. This met with not surrender of the attackers but with profound escalation—something any practitioner of the martial arts could have told me. I reflected; I tried to keep intuiting the right path of action; I searched for the Aikido master within. As the attacks continued, I tried the passive approach; I stopped responding to newspaper diatribes and media blitzes. Finally there was a review committee appointed by the chancellor of our campus to determine if we should be teaching TT in the school of nursing.

I was summoned to appear before the committee. Following my own advice and the popular wisdom of our time, I tried desperately to "let go of attachment to the outcome" of this review. I continued with my passive approach, and I affirmed every day that the outcome was not in my hands; that the process would unfold as it needed to; that all things change; that I could not know what should happen and that maybe the time for TT was

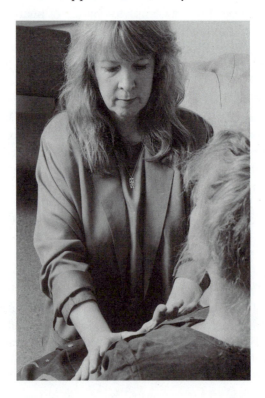

ending. I surrendered, I thought. But the more I tried to let go and surrender, the more deeply depressed I became. I felt as though I was dying but could not save myself. I had tried fighting fire with fire to no avail. I believed that surrender and letting go was the only option.

One day, only a week before my scheduled appearance before the committee, I had a sudden memory of a film on Mother Theresa which I had seen some years before. I remembered that when she was asked how she accomplished so much she answered that she did not, that God accomplished all things in her. When pushed for how that process actually worked, Mother Theresa elaborated. When there was an issue or a project to consider, she first took it to prayer. She did her best to discern what action needed to be taken—in her language, where she was called, or to what. Having discerned right action, she then did it 100%, no reservations, no second guessing. When she finished doing what she felt called to do, she surrendered the outcome to God—also 100%.

It hit me like a bolt of lightening—I was trying to surrender and let go before I had discerned and carried out right action in the situation. Passive ignoring of the media attacks might have been right action for that situation, but allowing the university review to proceed without any careful analysis from me was not. It became perfectly clear, and in four days I wrote a thirty page paper addressing the "academic relevance of Therapeutic Touch as a healing art in nursing." I prepared extensive appendices of the TT literature and other documentation to place TT squarely within the discipline, and brought a 100 page binder, with a table of contents on top, to each member of the review committee when I went to meet with them. The prepared table of contents served as an agenda and focused the discussion in our meeting.

When I left the meeting I felt triumphant, free, and ecstatic. Now I could let go. Now I could surrender to the unfolding mystery. Now that I had discerned what I needed to do and done it 100%, I could let go of attachment to the outcome of their view. Ultimately, the committee supported our academic freedom to continue teaching TT while acknowledging that we needed more research and that there was no scientific evidence for the existence of energy fields—our position exactly. What I learned is this: we can't truly let go of attachment to outcome until we've discerned as best we can what the situation is calling forth from us and then given it completely. Short of this, letting go of attachment to outcome can actually be a disguised form of anesthesia against our pain or an abdication of our responsibilities, choices that lead not to freedom but to death. When we stop acting in ways that are authentically ours, giving what is called for from the depths of who we are, something in us dies. What we need to let go of in order to be free is our demand that any given situation turn out the way we want it to. We do this while realizing that "letting go" is not a replacement for carefully considered, conscious action, and participation in the unfolding process, but rather the last step in that action.

This, then, is the source of our true healing power; the capacity to discern right action, the courage to do it, and the trust to let it go. Learning this, one somehow becomes less afraid, or less concerned about being afraid. As Audre Lorde said: "When I dare to be powerful, to use my strength in the service of my vision, then it becomes less and less important whether I am afraid." For me, at this juncture, that which calls me forth, which moves in me as the spirit of discernment and the courage of right action and the trust of letting go is nothing less than Love itself, the Divine Mystery. By grace I trust that we are becoming a better and better healing team.

Lynn Rew
RN, EdD, C, HNC, FAAN

Associate Professor, School of Nursing, The University of Texas at Austin, Editor, Journal of Holistic Nursing, Austin, Texas

My birth on October 29, 1943, in Washington, Iowa, was predicted with certainty by my mother. My maternal grandmother, Besse Swift Wittrig, was to celebrate her fiftieth birthday on that date and my mother, Clara Wittrig Cannon, was convinced that I would share her birthday. Mom's physician disagreed with her, but he could not hold me back and I entered the world, nee Donna Lynn Cannon, on the very date my mother had proclaimed. For the next thirty years, my "little grandma" (as she was affectionately known to my only brother, Max, and me) and I celebrated our birthdays together with an extended family. Those birthdays are among my fondest memories of a little grandma who was a perfect role model of gentleness and unconditional love.

My parents, Charles and Clara, were high school sweethearts who married without ever going to college. My father worked at a variety of different jobs until he took up farming before I was born. My mother was a homemaker and an expert seamstress who also had a beautiful soprano voice, which eventually led her to become a church choir director. Our nuclear family of four lived in the same rural community in southeastern Iowa until my brother and I went off to college and then married and pursued careers in other parts of the country. As a child growing up on a farm I was quickly exposed to the various miracles of life and death: the birth of piglets, the wonder of green cornstalks shooting through the dark earth, the delight of kittens and bunnies and lambs in the spring, the suffering of a bird with a broken wing, and the passing of a beloved dog who had finally lived life to the fullest. This stability of rural living and exposure to the realities of life provided a framework for understanding the unity of life and its importance in healing.

Throughout my childhood I was always going full speed ahead to explore the world and to try every new skill I developed. Because I was on a farm and far from other playmates, I made friends with many animals and had a rich fantasy life that included being a mother, a baker, a storekeeper, a secretary, a teacher, an artist, and a doctor. I dressed my kittens in doll clothes and pretended they were my babies and I made dozens of mud pies on the roof of the chicken house over the long summer afternoons. When my mother did the spring house cleaning, I pretended the piles of clothing were the merchandise I was selling in my general store. I saved envelopes and stamps so that I could have a well-equipped office to perform my secretarial duties. When I fantasized about being a teacher and an artist I drew diagrams on my chalkboard on the back porch or on the sidewalk behind our big farmhouse. But it was the dreaming that I would be a physician that captured my interest the most. My curiosity prompted me to perform many postmortem examinations on animals of various kinds and from this I learned basic anatomy and physiology. I also cared deeply about each of the animals who had passed on.

My childhood was characterized by the security of a loving family. My parents and grandparents were devout Christians and I remember hearing many conversations about how to help others who were less fortunate than us. These conversations were then transformed into actions that, as my father used to tell me, "speak louder than words." While my childhood was generally marked by love and security, it was punctuated by periodic injuries and illnesses (my own and others) from which I learned much about nursing and healing. I learned that unexpected injuries and serious illnesses brought families and communities closer together. I learned that while the doctor performed the amazing surgical procedures that knit bones together and removed a gangrenous appendix, it was the nurse who bandaged the wounds and soothed the pain and anxiety. I learned that chronic illness and birth anomalies made people strong and accentuated their uniqueness rather than weakening them and making them stand out as freaks. I learned that hot soup and crackers, a handful of garden flowers, gentle rocking, and prayer were all part of the healing process.

So many things about my childhood contributed to my identity as an adolescent. It was during my high school years that my aspirations turned from medicine to nursing. This was not because I had a burning desire to become a nurse, but because it seemed prudent and possible, given the other goals I had for my life: becoming a wife, a mother, and a responsible citizen. My first two years at college were some of the most exciting times of my life. I had dreamed of living in a city and of having friends with whom to do things. Learning the history of nursing, taking chemistry and microbiology, and studying anatomy and physiology at the university confirmed that I had chosen a noble profession. When I left the university after two years to marry my mate for life, dick (who prefers that his name be spelled with a lowercase 'd'), my father made us promise that I would finish my education. Five years later and ten days prior to the birth of our twins, Richard and Carina, I had completed my BSN at the University of Hawaii. I was on top of the world—I had it all—a handsome husband, two perfect babies, and a baccalaureate education. The first year as a new mother and nurse was to be one of the best educations of my life. Not only did I learn how to feed two screaming babies simultaneously, but I learned about pyloric stenosis, febrile convulsions, spica casts, patience, and organization. These skills would serve me well as I pursued my nursing career.

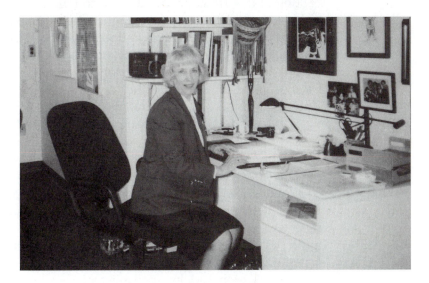

My first few years as a bedside nurse were not particularly remarkable. I honed my technical skills and improved my decision-making. I became more efficient and more empathic with my patients. But I was often frustrated by the lack of autonomy in my practice and the paucity of time I had to sit with my patients and their families and really get to know them and what they needed to feel better. The obvious answer to these frustrations was the pursuit of graduate education. In 1975 I received my MSN in Community Health Nursing from Northern Illinois University (NIU) and went right on to complete the EdD degree in Counselor Education from the same institution in 1979. While pursuing these degrees, I worked full-time as a nurse educator at Elgin Community College and part-time at NIU. Being a nurse educator was a challenge and, for the most part, it was fulfilling. In the last year of my doctoral program I proposed to a medical group in Woodstock, Illinois, that I could develop a department of health education and counseling. The purpose of this department would be to offer medical and surgical patients additional information and alternative therapies as adjuncts to the mainstream care they were receiving from the physicians. My proposal was accepted as a component of my education (a type of internship) and when it worked out well, the medical group invited me to stay as a full-time employee after completing my doctorate.

Working in this arena provided me with much of the flexibility and autonomy I had been longing for. I had time to read about innovative healing modalities and to test some of my ideas about the meaning of suffering and healing to people from all walks of life. It was during this phase of my career that I was invited to become a founding member of the American Holistic Nurses' Association (AHNA). It was wonderful to align my energy with that of many other nurses whose personal and professional journeys had brought us to a similar place in our understanding of the healing resources of nursing. These colleagues affirmed my beliefs and encouraged my pioneering efforts with my clients. These colleagues also challenged the limits of my beliefs and begged me to stretch even further in my quest for improving nursing practice and education.

In the past decade my personal and professional life styles have shifted once again. My children are grown and living independently as professional adults. My daughter has become a nurse and a dog-trainer (for wheelchair-bound individuals). My son is an attorney who specializes in employment law. My husband of 33 years is thinking about early retirement and I have just embarked on a postdoctoral fellowship in adolescent health at the University of Minnesota. Over the years I have felt that I missed something by not pursuing an education in medicine. Somehow being a nurse was only second-best. However, since I've been in this fellowship with colleagues who are physicians, psychologists, social workers, and nurses, I'm relieved to know that I probably followed what was the best path for me. This year away from my responsibilities as a faculty member at The University of Texas at Austin, I have had time to reflect and consider the importance of nursing in my life and in the lives of those around me. I have come to see that all the visions I had in my childhood fantasies are parts of who I am as a nurse healer: a mother, a baker, a storekeeper, a secretary, a teacher, an artist, and a doctor. To enter into the sacred temple of healing, one needs to be humble yet skilled. Humility allows us to recognize that it is not we who are doing the healing, but that as nurses or mothers or doctors or friends, we are merely the conduits for energy to pass through. We must use our skills in mothering, nurturing, keeping inventories, communicating, teaching, creating beauty, and administering treatments. Whatever talents and interests we have can be brought into this sacred place with us and are to be used as expressions of love and healing in every interaction with others.

To those nurses who wish to affirm themselves as healers, I would encourage you to remember the hopes and dreams of your youth. Allow yourself to be all that you can be because you never know when something as simple as a smile or as subtle as a gentle touch on an arm can be filled with healing energy. Healing is not about acquiring academic degrees, holding professional appointments, or applying specific technical skills. Healing is more about being than it is about doing. Healing is about being real and about being vulnerable. It's about feeling and thinking, touching and hurting, grieving and celebrating, wondering and knowing. And, above all, it's about being in harmony with all of creation.

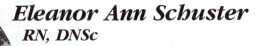

Eleanor Ann Schuster
RN, DNSc

Associate Professor, College of Nursing, Florida Atlantic University, Boca Raton, Florida

My mother was a nurse. I grew up observing "nurse type" actions, like improvising solutions to problems and making-do whatever the situation. She would take me to meet her classmates from her "training" years; once we went to the Home for the Incurable where she introduced me to friends she had cared for years before. She often shared her choice, colorful, and sometimes raunchy stories, like the night an orderly from her floor hid in a morgue drawer to frighten one of his co-workers who had a body to put away. I was encouraged to clean and dress my father's wounds if he cut himself while doing chores. I extended my ministrations to all, on one occasion wrapping an injured rat in a linen table napkin to provide comfort for him (or her). But nursing wasn't for me. I had other ambitions and entered a high school premed curriculum. That (medicine) was not to be once I discovered that cutting classes and general goofing off were much more engaging than studies. When college time came, I was not among the group of my friends who enrolled. My mother said she would not finance my irresponsible ways ("tough love" was not yet a term to describe her motivation). Diploma program nursing was one of very few viable options, so I began the program at St. Joseph's Hospital in Phoenix, Arizona. Earning my cap there was a turning point—I could succeed and I did. It was the first time I can remember being focused and deliberate, although I do not recommend this form of apprenticeship for today's nursing. I learned from the Sisters of Mercy some attitudes I still cherish—treating patients and families as honored guests, a willingness to attempt anything, a sense of community. When I moved to San Francisco, I learned something from the Jesuits at the University of San Francisco about the splendor and discipline of scholarship. It was 1955, and even then, head nurses were expected to have a baccalaureate degree so I went (albeit kicking and screaming) to "re-do" my nursing education. Through that experience, in the context of the vast cultural opportunities of the City, (as we called San Francisco), I began a teaching position. To sustain such a role, further education was needed by way of master's and doctoral work. With grounding in family/child nursing and many other enriching experiences, I embarked on teaching as a career. (I will admit here that I have had few goals in my life, and "teaching" was not one of them. For me, life unfolds as I take a particular path when opportunities become apparent.) About that time, another turning point came when I was told by a head nurse to do something else rather than continue to hold a dying two-year-old child. I did "what I was told," learning the next night that Bobby had died. I determined then never to permit institutional directives or anyone in authority to supersede what I saw as right for my practice of nursing. I had many experiences with major changes in health care, such as the first postanesthesia recovery rooms, the first ICUs, family centered maternity care, and the advent of contraception availability. It was all most interesting and invigorating, then and in current memory.

The notions of nurse as healer and holistic nursing did not enter my awareness all at once, and maybe they haven't yet. But I do know things that guide my practice:

1. Who I am is as important as what I do. This is a constant balancing. The only thing I can change is me and thus affect the collective in one way or another. For me, the healing way is working from the inside out.

2. I prefer to take myself lightly although I have my ponderous moments. For instance, at the post office, I sometimes request (in loud tone) some Lawrence Welk stamps. When they don't know what I mean I talk about equal opportunity. If there is an Elvis stamp, surely there should be a Lawrence stamp! I carry bubble liquid in my car so when I am stopped at a train track or a bridge, I roll down the window and blow bubbles. I know it amuses me and often the other people who are waiting in line.

3. No job is demeaning. Nursing, I believe, is honored to be present and nurturing through our astounding intimate access to all of life, a priestly role. We midwife, as men and as women, all of life's transitions.

4. My job, our job, I believe is to strive for "right relationship" with all being—environment, animals, the ugly, the beautiful, self, institutions—all being.

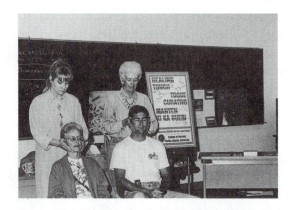

5. I ask each day for the strength and light to be part of all the turmoil and paradox of things, not just an onlooker.

6. I choose to live until I die and expect to leave this life with a whoop, not a whimper.

There is a poem that is mine, somehow. It is not meant to be understood at once or through conventional whim. It causes me to catch my breath yet it informs me. It says to me, among other things, that I am called to become simpler and clearer until I become Light, and so are we all.

The Desert Has Many Teachings

In the desert
Turn toward emptiness
Fleeing the self.
Stand alone
Ask no one's help
And you will quiet,
Free from the bondage of things.
Those who cling to the world
endeavor to free them,
Those who are
Care for the Sick,
But live alone
Happy to drink from the waters of sorrow
To kindle love's fire
With the twigs of a simple life.
Thus you will live in the desert.

–Adopted from a poem by Mechtilde of Magdeburg
(1210–1280 AD)

Donna Taliaferro
RN, PhD, CNS

*Assistant Professor, School of
Nursing, University of Texas
Health Science Center at San
Antonio, San Antonio, Texas*

I was born in Poplar Bluff, Missouri,
and raised in southern Missouri and
southern Illinois. My family was a traditional one with my mother a housewife
and my father superintendent of different
school systems. Both my parents supported lifelong learning and
today my father and mother continue with a multitude of endeav-
ors after many years of retirement.

When I was approaching my senior year in high school and
college was around the corner, I had many decisions to make.
During the late 60s and early 70s there were few choices we could
make. They were either teaching or nursing. I knew I didn't want
to be a teacher. Ironically, I have been teaching for the past fifteen
years. I started my journey as a volunteer at the local hospital. I
worked two evenings a week and some on the weekends as a
candy striper. I learned so much that I knew nursing was my path.
I started nursing school at the university and was hooked from the
first class. I always knew from the start that nursing was going to
be more than a job. It just fit. It was right for me. However, my journey in healing and caring didn't begin for many years. I became a
critical care nurse and very efficient in skills and technology. I was
so concrete in my thinking that I never allowed my mind to accept
another way of knowing. It was during my master's program that
I became exposed to theory based nursing practice and different
ways of thinking. Again, I didn't allow myself the opportunity to
open my eyes. What I did see was how we treated each other. As
I started teaching right out of my master's program, I continued to
see a pattern of lack of caring for one another. We were taught how
to care for patients but not how to care for ourselves and others.

The turning point in my career came in 1986 when my transformation to healing and caring began. I owe it all to Dr. Nancey
France. She and I had not started our doctoral programs yet. In

November that year we were driving to Florida from Kentucky to attend a National League for Nursing meeting. Suddenly she said "I have to make a phone call." We pulled off at the next place and she was gone for over twenty minutes. When she came back, I asked her what took so long and her response was "Oh, I was doing Therapeutic Touch (TT) for some football players." I told her I was driving the rest of the way—I thought she had lost her mind. However, that incident started a creative discussion on TT. Nancey had been teaching TT and practicing TT for several years. I knew she was weird, but I liked how she was with the world. She talked me into taking the course. I did, but my concrete thinking processes just couldn't accept this "energy thing." How could I rearrange someone else's energy?

The second pivotal point came when I attended the first annual Caring Conference a few months later. I was hooked. That was the piece that was missing. I could finally articulate what nursing was to me. Caring became the essence of nursing. Yes, we take care of patients. I don't mean the physicality of caring for a patient. I mean the moral, ethical, philosophical caring that comes from within your being. Caring is what opened my mind to all kinds of nursing interventions that are grounded in healing. TT was becoming a part of me. I still couldn't feel anything. It was months before I felt energy. Even though I couldn't feel anything, I still practiced TT. I was beginning to see results. I used it on plants, the dog, the hamster and yes, on my children. I liked what was happening. But what was happening more, was how I was emerging. I was changing inside. I needed more. As that old feeling surfaced on how nurses treat nurses, I began to see how caring needs to start with self. If you don't care for yourself first, you cannot care for others. I started teaching TT and caring. This is such a challenge to teach and practice caring in a world that devalues caring. Our world around us defuses the important piece that is unique to nursing. Health care has inhibited many of our caring modalities for financial profit. My struggle is how to impart that we must hang on to the uniqueness of nursing. The first thing I teach in my caring class is how to care for ourselves. Actually, I have difficulty believing I am a healer when the healing potential is in all of us. Some suppress it and others seem to flourish with it. I find such strength when I see that potential emerge in my students as they begin their journey in healing and caring. I never expect an outcome, therefore I am always surprised by the results.

This is such an exciting time for nursing. Since over one-third of all Americans are seeking alternative healing practices, the opportunities for nursing are endless. The integralness of caring to the practice of nursing has flourished in recent years. Holistic practice has taken on new meaning. Ann Boykin, Dean, School of Nursing, Florida Atlantic University, states that "caring is centered in authentic presencing where selfless sharing and fortifying support flourish and lead to uplifting consequences." One student said to me one day in class, "When I leave here I feel like I have been to church." What a wonderful uplifting consequence for me. I know that when I touch the lives of students, they touch someone else. What could be more healing than that?

I often wonder if caring can really be taught. Another student told me that caring isn't taught, it is caught. As nurses we have a moral obligation to model caring to each other and to our students and patients. Practice random acts of kindness and caring. I see this bumper sticker on many cars. In our world of violence and pain, it is sometimes difficult to be a caring person. It has to be worked on. For some it comes easy and for others we have to struggle to develop that potential. I hope that every student that I come in contact with leaves with the message that each one of us is caring in some way. Mother Theresa said "Kind words can be short and easy to speak but their echoes are truly endless." Words are very powerful but our actions speak louder.

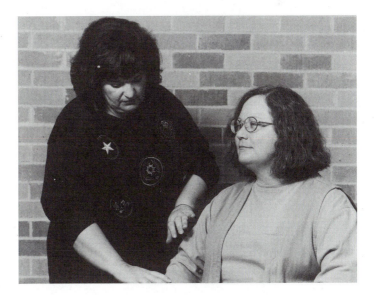

If I could leave you with one thought, it is to open your heart and your mind to new ways of being. The opportunity to develop a healing, caring potential is in all of us. There are so many rewards that come from living a caring based practice in your life and in your work. I can't begin to imagine the transformation of the world if we all developed the healing potential that lies within. Being a caring, healing person is not without risk. It opens our heart and our soul to new and different situations. Some may be painful and others so glorious that they overcome the painful ones. Strength and perseverance are necessary to continue the journey. Peace and harmony abound. If all of us followed the five Cs of caring (competence, confidence, compassion, conscience, and commitment) that were developed by Sister Roach, we would all become caring individuals. It is this philosophy that I try to live with my family, my colleagues, and my students. This is my journey in healing and caring.

Sharon Scandrett-Hibdon
RN, FNP, PhD, CHTP/I

Private Practice, Educator,
Aubrey, Texas

I was born in Indianapolis, Indiana, at the end of the Second World War to parents who had lived during the great depression. I came in as most babies, rather sensitive. My own awareness of emotions began when I was an infant. I recalled picking up my mother's anxiety breastfeeding. I noticed adults were having a difficult time. When my brother was born, I thought he was beautiful and I adored him. He was a very sick little boy who almost died of bronchial pneumonia. In spite of his rough start, I remember thinking how kids seemed more healthy than adults.

As a young child, I seemed to understand things, especially spiritual ideas in the Bible in an unusual way. I was somewhat surprised at these understandings as was my Sunday school teacher. A game I used to play with neighbor kids who were Catholic was being a "nun," even though I was a Methodist. I knew I loved very deeply and helped whenever I could. I always tried to assist animals as well. I loved plants and had my own small garden when I was young. I especially remember being fascinated by the huge black and yellow spiders that I saw in my garden on their beautiful webs.

When I decided to be a nurse I was a young girl in the Methodist Youth Fellowship with the commitment to be of service to God. I wanted to be a medical missionary. As a child I read about Tom Dooley and Albert Schweitzer and was inspired by their lives of service. My Methodist Youth Fellowship leader chided me for this statement of commitment saying it was just something I felt at the moment but would probably not manifest. I remember feeling hurt by her doubt. No one in my family claimed to be healers or interested in medicine. My mother used to faint when we kids would get hurt. But the fire of desire to serve burned brightly. I decided upon nursing without knowing too much about it. Being accepted at a diploma school of nursing and the University of Iowa even though I lived in Illinois, I was counseled by the dean of the diploma school to go to Iowa since the BSN was the wave of the future. So I did and I have been ever grateful for that angel which guided me in a sound direction.

My journey as a nurse has been a rich one. I began as a rotating staff nurse at the United States Public Health Hospital in San Francisco in 1965. After a year of Honeymooning in the golden gate city, my husband and I headed to Dallas where I taught nursing in a diploma school, Methodist School of Nursing, for two years. Then we moved to Houston where I went back to school in the Psychiatric-Mental Health nursing master's program at Texas Women's University. During this time I had my first son, Brad. Upon completion of my master's in nursing I went back to the University of Iowa and became an instructor at the University of Iowa on a part-time basis. In 1974 I left the College of Nursing to become a clinical nurse specialist in Iowa's outpatient psychiatric clinic. After my second son, Kelby, was born, I began to study for my PhD at the University of Iowa which I completed in 1980. I taught part time at the college while continuing as a clinical specialist. I moved to Memphis, Tennessee, after a divorce to create a metaphysical light center called Nexus and to teach at the University of Tennessee. I remained in Memphis for thirteen years. At the university I taught a popular elective called "Wholistic Nursing" for twelve years and attempted to integrate holism into the undergraduate curriculum.

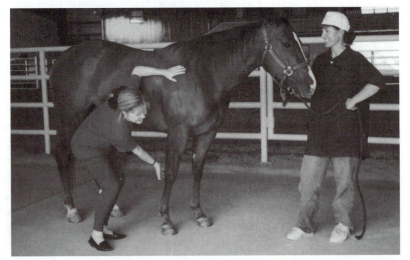

Where my challenge has come is working with groups of people to create a common vision, particularly in creating light centers. These efforts work with much enthusiasm for a period, then people move on to their next lesson. The transitions are always hard for the maintainers which is how I see myself. I am like a vessel holding the vision and light. I am a healer in that I create healing communities, first at Nexus which was a spiritual community outside Memphis, Tennessee. I moved to Memphis in order to create this light center with Lina Duckworth, Larry Berntsen (later Lina's husband), and Joe Simons. We blended with Karen Freeman, Francie and Nathan Atkeison, Emily Fox, and others to create a very clear center which lasted for more than thirteen years. Out of this effort was created a wholistic clinic entitled the Life Patterning Center which began as a collective integrated practice but then became an individual practice site in Memphis. Much education and healing was accomplished within these two creations.

I moved near Dallas in 1993 to assist Beverly McGregor and Don Strickland along with others to create The Health Institute. During this time I served as president of AHNA and went to school and completed my FNP at the University of Tennessee. I commuted from Texas to Memphis focalizing the master's program in psychiatric family nurse practitioner. So as you might guess, my plate was very full and I learned to focus only on each moment. The Health Institute was a monumental practice which took the basic philosophy of Life Patterning Center and attempted to create an integrated practice. This worked for a while under the direction of Beverly, however, management misguidance and inconsistencies were the downfall of this effort after three short years. My role in this was supportive, but mostly absent since I was teaching in Memphis and in the Healing Touch program. Plus I traveled a lot for AHNA and the office of Alternative Medicine as one of the program advisors on the first Council.

I have learned much by all of these paths. I have learned to trust myself and my commitment to whatever my vision is. I also have developed greater understanding and tolerance for others' paths. I know I am a good instructor and I hold the light well. I know my bliss is in the healing arts and science. I enjoy giving presentations to nurses about healing arts. All the while I continue to bring the healing energy into my work, whether it be as a psychotherapist, a family nurse practitioner in rural health, or as a healing touch practitioner or instructor.

My advice to others is that you always follow your dreams. It isn't always easy, but there is much richness and growth. Do what gives you bliss, rather than doing what you think you should. Follow your own path of your heart, rather than fulfilling others' dreams. I have been a risk taker and I have found my bliss. My growth has exploded forward by all that I have learned. Stand in your truth and be patient and gentle with yourself. I dream of a better world for us all; each of us brings a piece of the whole into each moment. May we all dance and sing along the way.

NURSES IN
ACUTE CARE

5

INTRODUCTION

Have you ever wondered about the personalities behind the faces of emergency department, critical care, or other acute care nurses? Lay persons often hold these practitioners in awe, thinking of them as highly skilled individuals who have helped them and their loved ones through the dramatic and traumatic times of crisis.

Hospital nurses were the primary practice group from the 1930s through recent times. However, during the early part of this century and now, once again, the shift has returned to care of the client in the home. The nurses who remain in hospital settings often specialize or become skilled in speciality areas due to continual updating of practice skills and increasing sophistication of acute care practice areas.

The nurses profiled in this section are representative of many other unnamed nurses who toil day after day, month after month to serve and to heal. They frequently work in an area of rapid client turnover and because of this, often have the briefest of encounters with their clients. These nurses are skilled not only in technological and psychomotor skills but also in the ability to make the most of the therapeutic moment.

Sandra Lutz
RN, MS, CFNP, CHTP/I

PRN Planned Parenthood, Private practice, Healing Touch Instructor, Perkins, Illinois

I was born, raised, and will probably be buried in central Illinois in a town called Perkins. I was born on April Fool's Day and the story is told that when the doctor told my father that I was a girl, my father thought it was an April Fool's joke. There was no burning desire to be a nurse while I was growing up. At one point, I was sure that I wanted to be a detective like Nancy Drew. Later, I felt I was destined to be a writer or a great actress. By the time I started high school, I was a little more practical and decided on secretarial work. I plunged into shorthand and typing with vim and vigor. However, as the years progressed, I didn't progress with any skill in typing or shorthand. After a stern lecture from the typing teacher, I came to the realization that secretarial work was definitely not my calling.

What was my calling? Here I was, a senior in high school, and I had no idea where I was headed or what I was fit for. One night as I lay in bed, I prayed fervently for God to show me what I was supposed to do. I woke up the next morning with the answer. It was very clear to me that I was supposed to go into nursing.

I imparted this news to my family. My mother was thrilled. She had a vested interest in the medical profession since she had been sick most of my tender years. I had no idea where I would go for this profession or what it entailed, but I was very sure that this was my calling. There were two schools of nursing right in the area, but I opted to get away from home and attend Lutheran Hospital School of Nursing in St. Louis. Looking back now, I wonder how different things might have been if I had gone to school in this area.

I had been going steady with my high school sweetheart, Gene, for two years. He wasn't happy about me going so far away to school. I felt a little torn too. I had a dream a couple of times that summer before going away to school. I was walking down the aisle to get married. I would just about get to the altar then I would stop and shout "I can't get married. I have to finish school!" It was part of the rules of nursing schools at the time, in 1955, that you couldn't be married and attend school.

Nursing was wonderful. I loved everything about it. The only area that I didn't enjoy was surgery. The first year went by quickly. It was all new and exciting. During the second year I started feeling the conflict between nursing and nesting. Gene had a good job and was making enough money to support a wife. It was getting harder and harder to say good-bye and go back to school (when I was able to make the trip home). I told my parents that I would like to quit school and get married. My mother responded by having a dinner and inviting Gene's folks in. I thought it was to discuss the possibility of marriage, but instead the four of them collaborated to try and convince us that we were too young, it would never last, I should finish school, and on and on. We had run into a brick wall. I went back to school like a good little girl.

A few months later, we took matters into our own hands. Gene came down to St. Louis one weekend and we eloped to Hernando, Mississippi. We were married in Hemando's Little Wedding Chapel. Gene took me back to school at the end of the weekend. We were married, but afraid to tell our parents, so we kept it a secret for the next four months. I was coming home for a month's vacation before I was to start my psychiatric rotation. I wasn't looking forward to this rotation, spending three months, most of it locked up, in the sanitarium. So, when I went home for vacation, I packed up everything and went home for good. Gene's mother cried for days, and my mother just looked at me and said "You know you can't come home again."

The nesting instinct had won temporarily, and for the next few years, I was busy having babies and making a home for our ever increasing family. During these years, I would continue to have the same recurring dream that I was back in nurses' training. At one point, with five children at home, I looked into the program at the local junior college. They had started an Associate Degree in Nursing and it was okay to be married. I talked with Gene and the kids about my going back to school. To my dismay the oldest son, Eric, became almost hysterical because I would be gone during the day. "What if I need you!" he cried. So I put my plan back on the shelf for a few more years. The dreams continued.

One night, I was sitting in the emergency room with my son, Matt, who seemed to be accident prone. As I watched the nurses bustling about taking care of patients, the conviction began to grow in me that this work was what I needed to be doing. The more I thought about it the more excited I became. When I got home, I talked it over with Gene. He thought it would be a good idea; I would have something to fall back on if anything ever happened to him. I found out later—he hadn't intended that I should actually go to work. The time was right. Our seventh child would be starting first grade in the fall, and the oldest one was in high school. Once I started school, the recurring dreams stopped.

I had been part of a weekly meditation group at that time. When I talked about my plans to the group, one of the women in the group, Sharon, said that she had quit nurses' training and got married, too. She decided to go back to school with me. It was wonderful to have a support person in this venture. We were two matrons entering the world of education surrounded by youngsters.

We had families to care for and houses to keep up while trying to fit in time for study and homework. There was many a night that found me trying to read or do my homework at 2 A.M. because there hadn't been the time or the quiet for me to do it until the family was in bed. I remember one morning I was trying to do some last minute cramming for a test we were going to have that day. Eric asked me to iron a shirt for him. I told him I was studying and he could do it himself (he knew how). His reply was "Well, I didn't know you gave up being a Mother!" Kids really know how to get to you!

The day of graduation finally came. The family was all there and very proud of my accomplishment. My Aunt Sharon congratulated me and told me I should look into holistic nursing. She had attended a workshop presented by Norman Shealy and felt that this would be the future of medicine. Unfortunately, in 1977, no one in central Illinois had heard anything about holistic health or holistic nursing.

It was she who actually precipitated my journey into the healing arts, by giving me the gift of a workshop entitled "Touch for Healing, A natural health care therapy." We went to the workshop together and that is where I was introduced to Dolores Krieger's work in therapeutic touch. During the workshop, we worked on each other. I discovered a cold spot over Sharon's elbow. I practiced sending energy as we were taught. Sharon told me later that she had problems with that elbow and had even had cortisone shots in it. The cortisone shot had left her ring and little finger numb. After I worked on her, the feeling came back in her fingers and her elbow never bothered her again. Needless to say, I ordered Dr. Krieger's book *Therapeutic Touch.*

I read the book, practiced on my friends and family, and yearned for a workshop that would be close enough for me to attend. I joined the American Holistic Nurses' Association, and received notices of workshops, but they were all too far away. Finally, there was one that was only an hour away by car. Janet Macrae, RN, PhD, was the workshop presenter, and the workshop was a wonderful experience. For the first time, I was with a whole group of people that talked my language. Since that first class, I have gone on to take other workshops in Therapeutic Touch. I found the Healing Touch workshops offered through AHNA to be a real growth experience for me. At first, I wasn't even going to take the classes. I had been doing Therapeutic Touch for ten years, why would I need to take the Healing Touch? However, I found the Healing Touch program challenged me and pushed me to expand my horizons.

I had continued my practice of Therapeutic Touch in whatever area of nursing I happened to be working. However, I was

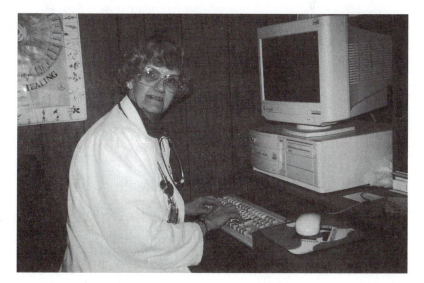

usually low key with it as central Illinois was not very open-minded about alternative therapies. In fact, at one point in my career, I was ordered to stop the "Voodoo." Since I have gone through the certification process with Healing Touch, I have more confidence in my credibility and can be more open with what and who I am. There are still many challenges to overcome in the use of Healing Touch in the central Illinois area, but there is support now from nurses who have taken the Healing Touch classes. There has also been more coverage in the media on alternative therapies.

I feel it is very important in nursing to be continually learning. That is probably why I have continued my education until I had my Master's Degree in Nursing. Many programs are now available in the healing arts and I continue to explore these. My advice to anyone pursuing a nursing career these days is to be open-minded and visionary. Dare to be different and creative. Nursing is still developing as a science, and as holistic nurses we can impact this development because we are a large collective of like minded individuals.

Joan Vitello-Cicciu
RN, MSN, CCRN, CS, FAAN

*Acting Nurse Manager Emergency
Department, Boston Medical
Center, East Newton Campus,
Boston, Massachusetts*

I was born in Boston, to Italian-Leban-
ese parents. I have lived here most of
my life except when I attended graduate
school at the University of Alabama in
Birmingham. I also see myself as an actor on
the great stage of life playing such everyday roles as wife, mother,
grandmother, and nurse. Other roles I engage include daughter (in-
law), sister (in-law), aunt, teacher, editor, consultant, speaker, writer,
facilitator, mentor, colleague, steward to professional organizations,
doctoral student, and friend.

Why did I become a nurse? It was 1966, the Vietnam War
was raging. I was graduating from high school and was headed
to college for a premedical major in biology. Within several
months of entering premed, I had lost my passion for school. I
found myself in a fiercely competitive environment. I was one of
three female students in a predominantly male environment and
not favorably looked upon by my classmates. Often I would hear
that I was taking up a seat that some male student should have
had! Unfortunately, this was a time when females were not welcomed in the halls of academia.

In my second year of college, I dropped out to get married
and had my daughter within the year. After her birth, I stayed home
for the first year gaining confidence in my role as a mother. When
Renee was sixteen months I went to real estate school and became
a real estate broker. I worked for four years as a broker and inte-
rior decorator. After working these years in business, I felt a void.
I yearned for more meaningful work. Feeling this void, I sought out
career counseling. I scored high in the social sciences and then did
some soul searching. I wanted a career where I could be in service
to human beings while maintaining a balance in my life. I chose a
career in nursing. I brought with me to the nursing profession my
values of caring, collaboration, commitment, and communication.

What do I hope to accomplish as a nurse healer? My nursing career began for a one month brief rotation on a vascular unit before embarking on my lifetime career in critical care. I started on a respiratory care unit and then quickly moved into a medical ICU. From there I worked as a clinical nurse in coronary care, surgical ICU, and a respiratory ICU. After six years as a clinician, I moved into a critical care unit instructor position and then pursued a graduate degree. Upon graduation with a master's degree in nursing, I began my journey as a critical care clinical nurse specialist. This remains the role I have been in for the last fourteen years.

When I initially began my nursing career, one important emphasis as a nurse healer was on meeting the physiological, psychosocial, and spiritual needs of patients and their loved ones. After all I went into nursing to care for the whole patient—the body, mind, and spirit. This focus came from my prior business practice of always trying to meet my customers' needs. As a nurse, I believed that I must value what patients and their loved ones were experiencing as a result of the disease or illness.

My masters' thesis reflected that belief when I explored the perceptions of patients having been administered pancuronium bromide while incubated in critical care unit. This belief was also the driving force with Dorothy, a 43-year-old woman with end-stage cardiac disease. Dorothy was tied to monitors, pumps, and tubes in the Surgical Intensive Care unit where I was the Clinical Nurse Specialist. It became apparent in my interactions with Dorothy that she was clinging to life until she could see her first grandson once again. This was in 1988 when visiting hours were so very restricted and I believed not conducive to helping patients to heal. I insisted that we break this rule and give this last gift to Dorothy. It was worth it. Once Dorothy saw him she had a peaceful look come over her and died the next day. My own personal meaning guided me because I was a new grandmother just like Dorothy. I instinctively knew what it meant for Dorothy to hold and feel that healing touch of her grandson that held such precious meaning for her.

Interestingly what I have hoped to accomplish as a nurse healer is what I hope to accomplish as a person, and that is to know myself and love myself; to know my limitations and to know my strengths; to always seek ways to bring out my full potential within myself; to keep in balance and to continue to nourish my physiological, psychological, and spiritual needs and to achieve the same for patients and their loved ones; and to know that my power is within and to be good to myself as well as my patients and their loved ones.

I truly believe that the healing begins within myself, by awaking my consciousness and embodying what I perceive as a better way to be and then taking control of my life through my actions. We can only heal the world around us by healing the world within us. I am truly committed to making this a better world by making myself a better person. My vision is of a world inhabited by healthy people that can reach their full potential through the integration of the body, mind, and spirit.

I would like to share a quotation with you that has helped me to overcome the obstacles and toxins in my life. It is by Dawna Markova, PhD.

> I will not die an unlived life
> I will not live in fear of falling
> or catching fire.
> I choose to inhabit my days
> to allow my living to open me,
> to make me less afraid, more accessible,
> to loosen my heart until it becomes a wing
> a torch, a promise
>
> I choose to risk my significance, to live
> so that which came to me as seed
> goes to the next generation as blossom
> and that which came to me as blossom goes
> on as fruit.

Wendy Wetzel
RN, MSN, FNP, HNC

*Nurse Practitioner, A Woman's Place,
Flagstaff, Arizona*

Holistic nursing has been the anchor that has kept me in this profession. At a time when I considered leaving nursing, I realized that my dissatisfaction came from the nonexpression of my beliefs as a holistic nurse. As I embraced all my convictions, I found new doors opening and old ones closing.

In June 1996, I celebrated my Silver Jubilee, twenty-five years of being a registered nurse. It was Father's Day, 1971, my graduation from a diploma program in the heart of the Midwest, and as my family looked on, the dean pinned our school pin on my fresh white uniform. As I looked into her face, I felt both joy and fear; joy at achieving a life dream, and fear at stepping into the world of professional nursing.

I recalled numerous confrontations with that very dean, who at one time told me that I would never finish the program, never pass my boards, and certainly not stay in the profession. She and I had had numerous challenges during my student days. I would challenge her beliefs and assert my understanding; she would return with threats and predictions of my certain failure. Now, on Graduation Day, I wondered if her prophecies would come true.

I had always wanted to be a nurse. According to family legend, I made this decision before my tenth birthday. I voraciously read everything I could on nursing, the biographies of Clara Barton and Florence Nightingale, the Cherry Ames series, even my mother's Red Cross manual on home nursing. I adored television series that focused on medicine: Ben Casey, Dr. Kildare, and Hennessey were weekly events. As my world expanded, my reading increased and I began planning my education and career. I was enthralled with the romance and mystery of medicine. My vision of nursing was far from the reality I would later experience, but the dream was constant and drove me forward. There was a knowing, deep inside, that nurses could and would change the world.

I began my formal education at the University of Wisconsin at Oshkosh where grades were inversely proportionate to the alcohol intake of the student. But as one of 400 applicants for 35 spaces in their brand new BSN program, I felt overwhelmed and with little chance of being selected. Rather than face the disappointment of being rejected, I applied to a hospital based program in Madison and was immediately accepted. In spite of the dean's predictions, I graduated, passed my boards, and immediately moved halfway around the world to the Republic of the Philippines with my Air Force husband.

At the Air Force Hospital at Clark AB, and under the wing of a passionate and caring head nurse, I honed my skills and moved into confidence as a professional. I was officially attached to the obstetrics unit, but often floated to other units, including the intensive care and surgical units, flight line, and emergency room. It was an initiation by fire, to care for wounded men from the Vietnam War, to see their young bodies peppered with shrapnel, or with limbs missing. It took me many years to even admit that this was my entry point into the world I had only gazed into before.

Once back in the states, I worked in neonatal intensive care and later pediatric orthopedics. While working with children, I had my first experiences with the human energy field. On the night shift in the nursery, I often found myself touching the babies and not just for nursing tasks. Often I held them, inside their isolettes, and felt their energy fields. One night, while caring for an especially sick neonate, I felt a shift of energy and if I knew then what I know now, would say that I felt and saw the baby's spirit begin to leave the physical body. There was a pink glow to the otherwise cyanotic infant and as its heart rate began to slow, I whispered "It's OK to go now." The pink seemed to rise above the child, hovering for a moment before it vaporized. Within a few moments, the heart beat slowed even more and finally stopped. We had been instructed not to resuscitate this child, for its degree of prematurity and other physical problems were insurmountable. So instead of providing heroic efforts at life support, I simply held the dying baby, easing its way out of this world and into the next.

In spite of enjoying pediatrics, my heart was in women's health care. To bridge the gap between my job and my heart, I became a Lamaze instructor and there I found the articulation of my belief that the mind, body, and spirit were linked and could not be separated. I began teaching Lamaze techniques even to those who were not pregnant, utilizing relaxation and imagery for stress reduction in many different situations.

My quest continued. I became a mom and while my son was young, continued my reading and learning, expanding my knowledge to oriental medicine, energetic healing, and nutrition. But when I returned to the working world, I found it difficult to integrate this information into the mainstream world of medicine and nursing. It was only after proving my nursing ability that I began to quietly interject my holistic perspective into my practice. I remember more than one occasion where the doctors, who could not openly acknowledge that I was holistic in perspective, simply turned their backs and told me to do whatever needed to be done.

I was truly "in the closet" in those years, not admitting professionally what I believed personally. I took classes, read books, listened to tapes, and sought alternative health care for myself and my child, but could not find the way to explain my beliefs to my co-workers and colleagues. While I learned a great deal about myself, I found myself feeling on the outside looking in. I called myself "holistic" but had little idea what that meant and certainly had no operational definition to share.

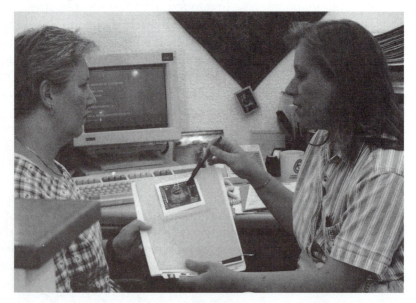

A tiny ad in the *American Journal of Nursing* led me to the American Holistic Nurses' Association, and I proudly say that my life has never been the same. At first, it was the safe haven I had been looking for, the collegial support of like-minded nurses and friends, and an arena in which I could walk my talk. It became, and still is, my family.

It was in graduate school that I finally found the courage of my convictions and "came out" for all the world to see. In the context of my nursing theory class, I found the support to talk about my beliefs and found acceptance for who I am. My theory paper "The Energy of Nursing" brought all my ideas to the printed page and made them seem more real for me.

Since those explosive years of self-identification and realization, I have focused my nursing skills in the area of women's health. I consider myself a holistic nurse practitioner and seek to walk between the worlds of allopathic and complementary medicine and nurse. I know that these worlds can and will be brought together. At first, I had to prove my skill as a nurse before introducing the holistic nature of my profession. But now, I share all of me, and most importantly, the holistic perspective that guides my practice.

My focus in women's health has led me to a private practice in Flagstaff, Arizona where I see clients in all phases of their lives. I was hired for my holistic philosophy as well as my skills in alternative and complementary care. I have come full circle within my own body, mind, and spirit and offer that perspective as a holistic nurse practitioner.

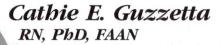

Cathie E. Guzzetta
RN, PhD, FAAN

Director, Holistic Nursing Consultants,
Nursing Research Consultant, Parkland
Memorial Hospital and Children's Medical
Center of Dallas, Dallas, Texas

Throughout history, master weavers have described the weaving of a tapestry as a calling, as transformation, as healing, or as a sacred work. The early, single threads of my tapestry have taken on new meaning over time as I have become clearer in mind and spirit about my mission of bringing holism and healing to the forefront of nursing. What follows are some of the threads that have been woven into my holistic tapestry.

THE EVOLVING TAPESTRY

When I was fresh out of school in the early 1970s, I worked in the intensive care unit. Having no experience, my nursing practice relied on book learning, rules, and regulations. The threads of my tapestry were primarily green.

I was hungry to master the pathophysiology of cardiac disease, hemodynamic monitoring, pharmacology, and the exploding critical care technology. Despite my hunger, I encountered disturbing events that conflicted with my logic and knowledge. I encountered patients like Mr. Verde, for example, who had been experiencing excruciating chest pain for hours one evening. While administering another IV dose of morphine sulfate, and desperate to help him, I instructed the patient to breathe deeply and relax. He screamed at me saying it wasn't that simple. I also remember, while visiting Mr. Noir for some preoperative coronary artery bypass surgery teaching, that he confided he was scared to death that he was going to die the next day. I said "Don't worry —try to relax—you'll be OK." The next morning the patient died on the operating table. Likewise, I remember caring for Mrs. Blanco who informed me that she survived her cardiac arrest the night before because of me. Looking puzzled, I asked her what she meant. She replied "Last night, I saw everything that was going on. The thinking-feeling part of me was getting ready to leave the room, but I felt a tap on my shoulder, turned around, saw you—and I knew I had to come back." I said something therapeutic like "Oh, I see" and never shared the conversation with anyone.

All of these clinical events became tightly woven into my tapestry. Despite returning to school to pursue a master's degree to obtain the missing knowledge base I thought I needed, something was still missing. Perhaps it was the biomedical contradictions I continued to encounter at the bedside. Perhaps it was the many times I observed how a patient's psychologic response to illness seemed to get in the way, inhibiting recovery, interfering with healing, and sometimes even causing death. Ultimately, I sensed that identifying and treating physical problems with body-oriented therapies was only half the answer. I realized I did not possess the knowledge and skills necessary to provide the body-mind-spirit care my patients needed.

Somewhere during this period, the composition of my tapestry changed. I found myself on a journey to discover my own wholeness and my path as a nurse healer. The journey demanded that I reexamine traditional beliefs and teaching that I had taken for granted and trust the wisdom that was unfolding. Two of my mentors, a nurse-physician team, Barbie and Larry Dossey, shared this journey with me. Together, we examined holistic models of health that acknowledge the interconnections of the body-mind-spirit. We searched for scientific documentation to validate the profound devastating effects, as well as the enormous healing effects, of consciousness on the body. We wrestled to unravel the assumptions of the holistic model to transform such concepts into concrete implications for bedside practice. We learned and personally experienced biobehavioral interventions such as relaxation, meditation, biofeedback, and imagery. We also listened intently to the healing stories of our patients.

The next step involved learning to combine the best of conventional critical care therapies with breathing exercises, head-to-toe relaxation scripts, imagery, biofeedback, and music. Because there were no textbooks, no mentors, and no schools to impart these strategies, we slowly began to incorporate such techniques into our daily bedside practice. Then we began to write and lecture about our experiences—squarely placing the philosophy, theory, research, and bedside techniques associated with holism into our articles, books, presentations, and research.

As our understanding of holism and healing continued to grow, we conceptualized holism as a paradigm for all of nursing's caring-healing practices: the very roots of professional nursing. We understood the concept of healing to be an ongoing process of becoming whole to finding meaning and purpose in life. We envisioned the role of a nurse healer as someone who embodies the scientific skill and spiritual commitment necessary to understand that healing is much more than curing disease. We defined a nurse healer *not* as an individual who cures *disease* (i.e., the pathophysiologic breakdown of the body), but rather as a guide who facilitates healing in the person with an *illness* who is also struggling with the symptoms, suffering, and consequences of disease to find the understanding, meaning, and wholeness embodied in the experience. It is from this insight we understood that although many patients cannot be—or chose not to be—cured, they all are in need of healing.

Twenty-five years later, the hues and shades of my tapestry have become fuller and richer as I have learned to blend my roles as a clinician, teacher, mentor, researcher, and author. Some of these threads are illustrated below.

Mr. Lavendera was having excruciating chest pain that he described as a tight, steel coil wrapped around his chest. As I injected the morphine into his IV line, I described what I was doing. I helped him shift his fast, chest wall breathing to slower, deeper, diaphragmatic breaths and suggested that he relax his tight fists and tense jaw. I recommended that he imagine the morphine going into his vein and straight to the source of his chest pain . . . seeing those powerful morphine molecules . . . unwrapping and loosening the tight, steel coil around his chest. Within minutes of using this multimodal therapy, Mr. Lavendera's heart rate returned to normal and he fell asleep.

Mr. Ruby told me that he was "scared to death" about his upcoming coronary angiography. I listened carefully to his story and the images he described. I then guided him in a relaxation and music therapy session and arranged for him to take music tapes, a recorder, and headphones to the catheterization laboratory. Following his catheterization, he said, "I was still scared but

I felt I had some control over the situation. I had something that *I* could do to help the procedure go smoothly and control my stress."

I mentored a team of emergency room nurses through an intense, two-year struggle to develop a research study investigating the effects of family presence during cardiopulmonary resuscitation and invasive procedures in the emergency department. When we began the project, it was filled with emotions, uncertainty, and risk. The project required changing conventional mindsets and longstanding rules. We did not know if we would ever carry out the study; some colleagues told us that this research would never be conducted at our institution. As the months dragged on and barriers were encountered, the team became discouraged. Yet, I sensed their passion and belief that the study was important and could make a difference in the lives of families and their loved ones. The motivation to continue became more focused as the team recognized how the study exemplified several fundamental principles of holism and healing. It illustrated the holistic imperative to preserve the wholeness, dignity, and integrity of the family unit from birth to death. It demonstrated that holistic care does not require any elaborate, alternative intervention but, as in the case of this study, simply requires the caring intent to "be with" and support another in the family presence experience. Ultimately, the study affirmed the belief that even during devastating illness, crisis, and death, healing can take place and growth toward wholeness can occur. In the end, the study received funding and is currently underway.

INTERCONNECTED TAPESTRIES

Tapestries are created by an intermeshing, intertwining, and connecting of individual threads configured by the weaver's consciousness and spirit. Each of the threads woven in my life tapestry has engendered a more vivid, dynamic, and deeper personal understanding about the nature of holism and healing and its explicit implications for nursing practice. Each of us, however, weaves our own tapestry to connect with the body-mind-spirit tapestry of others. Weaving a great tapestry is usually a collective effort; it is not often done in isolation. In the search for meaning and purpose in my work and life movement, the inseparable threads of my tapestry have interconnected with others in the healing journey toward wholeness.

* Abridged from: C.E. Guzzetta, Weaving a Tapestry of Holism. *J Cardiovasc Nurs* August, 1997 (In press).

Jill Strawn
RN, MSN, CS

Doctoral Candidate, Columbia University, New York Adjunct Faculty, School of Nursing, College of New Rochelle, New Rochelle, New York

I was born and raised until eleven years old in Quakertown, Pennsylvania, a small town where my mother's family had lived for several generations. I knew I wanted to be a nurse early in my childhood and would follow our family doctor around whenever he came to visit. I was the only girl child, with one younger and two older brothers. My father had epilepsy which was never well controlled and never named for me until I was sixteen. However, his petit mal seizures were evident and in some ways the cause of a family tragedy which precipitated a move from Pennsylvania to Long Island.

The move had wonderful consequences for me in that I was thrown into a better school system where I was encouraged to think of a career for myself and where my grades enabled me to receive a state scholarship for higher education. I don't think I ever considered any other option than nursing—I wanted to help people. Although I had hoped to attend a collegiate nursing program, my parents wanted more "protection" for me, so I went to an Episcopal diploma school in New York City, St. Luke's Hospital School of Nursing.

In 1967, as I was about to graduate, the ANA announced its recommendation for the baccalaureate degree as minimum qualification for professional nursing and I took it to heart. I enrolled in Hunter College as soon as I finished St. Luke's. However, those were the days before there were qualifying exams for exemption from basic courses and I was devastated to be informed that I would receive only one year of credit for my three years. I wasn't about to repeat all that work and so transferred into the political science department and had a terrific time broadening my horizons. For a while I seriously considered leaving nursing for law, which seemed in keeping with my new sense of empowerment.

I did well on the LSAT exam, but by then was working in an out-patient inner city clinic where I saw a different kind of nursing role, the public health nurse. These were feisty women who were politically active and seemed empowered in their community practice. It made me realize there might be more options in nursing than I had been exposed to at St. Luke's where I had trained and worked all through college.

I started to tune into the death and dying movement which was just burgeoning and I realized that I wanted to find a role where I could counsel seriously ill and dying individuals and their families. I knew I would need more education in mental health and that meant a master's degree in Psychiatric Mental Health Nursing. I had my first experience of feeling a divine guidance when the only graduate nursing school that allowed nonnursing baccalaureate applicants and that had one of only two psychiatric liaison programs in the country accepted me in 1975.

The desire to counsel people with physical illness was the beginning of my starting to put people back together again, to understand how emotions influence and are influenced by phys-ical illness. When I finished my MSN and got my first clinical spe-cialist position in a hospital in Philadelphia, the city was a hot-bed of holistic health education. Through opening to this bur-geoning new paradigm, I found a spiritual focus that helped me make sense of the suffering I witnessed in my work and which has sustained me personally and professionally ever since. I took advantage of training opportunities in hypnosis and therapeutic touch and started to incorporate them in my practice. I became a regular attendee at Pumpkin Hollow Farm where Dolores Krieger and Dora Kunz held forth in the summer. I got to know other nurses who were on a similar path and I joined the TT organiza-tion, The Nurse Healers' Professional Association, Inc.

Part of my job role at Jefferson Hospital was to offer con-tinuing education to staff nurses. This nursing environment encouraged creativity, so I developed and ran workshops in holis-tic health and body/mind therapies. Teaching became a major vehicle for the expression of my healing philosophy and has remained consistently so over the past fifteen or so years. In 1981 I took a job at Yale School of Nursing in the program from which I graduated. I started a Therapeutic Touch study group for the stu-dents and was an advisor for the first master's thesis on that topic at that school. I edited two issues of *Holistic Nursing Practice*, one on "Rehumanizing the Acute Care Environment" and the other,"Healing AIDS."

I suppose the most amazing spiritual discovery I've had along the way has been the calling to do AIDS work. I was a reluctant participant in the care of the first AIDS patient at Yale New Haven Hospital in 1983 and was gradually pulled by the heartstrings into the most meaningful work I could ever hope to find. At some point, after it became clear that this work had chosen me, rather than the other way around, I also realized that all the previous experience in psychiatric liaison nursing with people with other life-threatening illnesses had been preparation for caring for people with HIV/AIDS.

Once I got past my own fears of contagion and stigma, I was ready to steadily become involved in the many aspects of supporting people with this terrible illness. As I gave more and more of myself, I received more also. As my heart led me, personal and professional blossoming followed. As I became involved with community activism, community education, professional writing, and speaking, I was able to bring a whole person perspective to each endeavor. I became a proponent of complementary therapies for people with HIV, writing and speaking about it off and on for many years, and creating a program integrating naturopathic medicine and therapeutic massage into HIV care in the community health center where I coordinated HIV mental health services.

The only obstacle to promoting and pursuing the kind of healing beliefs and practices that attract me is my need to be accepted and embraced by those who doubt the validity of such work or actively devalue it. That desire ebbs and flows. In the last several years the environment in Connecticut has become more accepting of complementary therapies and there has been a resurgence in interest and enthusiasm that has supported my work.

That brings me to what I'd like to share with other nurse healers. It's easier to grow and flourish when you have some kind of support—a friend, colleague, or group of like-minded individuals who will encourage you in pursuing your calling.

Rita L. Kluny
RN, BSN

Neonatal and Pediatric Critical Care
Nurse, New Orleans, Louisiana

Illness has been a regular component in my life for as long as I can remember. Someone in my family, including myself, was always sick, in pain, or having surgery. Financial pressures, and emotional and physical abuse added to the intensity of my childhood. From a very early age, I took care of someone.

My first experience in nursing occurred at age 13. I was admitted for surgical correction of a quite severe curvature of the spine. In the week before I was casted, I helped the short-staffed nurses. I handed out juices, and fed and played with the children who were unattended. I waited on those who were bed bound. I loved most of the nurses. In the weeks ahead, when I was suffering in bed, they were very kind, patient, and compassionate. Their attention was very healing to me. There was one nurse there, though, that scared me. She was angry all the time. My experience with her served me well to understand how a nurse's personality could infuse a patient's spirit with hope or with fear.

The pain and growth of that yearlong process in bed sparked my passion to be of service to people. I was fortunate to receive a full scholarship from the state for my BSN at the University of Pittsburgh. I was a natural at the bedside. I knew what being a patient was; I understood pain. I worked part-time as a nurse technician. My job was a sharp contrast to the ideals of the nursing program at school.

The obstacle I faced was to constantly be in pain. I suffered silently. Lifting adults made it worse. I took a lot of aspirin, but my greatest medicine was my sense of humor. Two weeks after graduation, I had my right kneecap surgically removed for chondromalacia. Emotionally and physically, this recovery was more difficult. I was angry. My friends were getting jobs as new grads and I was at home again, which felt very confining after experiencing independence. In defiance, I would go dancing on my crutches. What I discovered was that my pain went away when I moved to the music.

My first job as a professional nurse was in Boston in pediatrics. I loved children, but I quickly became disheartened. My assignments consisted of either eight babies or twelve toddlers—all unattended, because back then, visiting hours were strictly limited to several hours each day. I ran from one to another and usually felt out of control. I lost my resilience with the constant urgency and resulting stress. I transferred into critical care. There, the nurses "ate their young." I learned a lot, but I needed a break, so I decided to travel. My family had never taken a vacation, so I wanted to be different.

I journeyed through Europe, then overland to the Far East. My exposure to many cultures awakened an awareness that I never expected. I sat in on philosophic discussions, and vicariously experienced the stories of other travelers who were seekers. I felt the presence that particularly emanated from one Buddhist nun in Nepal and a Buddhist monk in Burma. I witnessed a chanting ceremony in a temple that brought me peace. It contrasted the heaviness of the religion of my childhood. I liked this version of God—it made more sense to me. My experience in these seven months birthed the concept of spirituality for me.

Travel was now in my blood. I joined the Peace Corps and spent two years in Costa Rica as a public health nurse in a jungle clinic. I became an integral part of a tiny community. My nursing became more holistic with new awareness of that concept. I realized that hospital nursing is so isolated from the family and the whole picture of their life. I visited patients in their homes. Initially, the sparse conditions surprised me. They lived with so little. I frequently saw the little medication packets that I dispatched (usually for parasites) sitting somewhere, unopened. I never understood why they wouldn't take care of themselves, and it frustrated me. It was a tough job that I loved and hated. I knew I would never change them. So why was I there? It took me years to realize that my greatest gift to these people was that I treated them as my equals, and that inadvertently, my behavior gave them an experience of dignity that they never forgot. What I learned from the Costa Ricans was the joy of simple living. They were happy people with richness of spirit despite their material poverty. I gave away a lot of possessions when I left.

In the year following this experience, I gave myself the gift of going to South America. In the Andes while alone and contemplating, I experienced an intense heightening of awareness. The insights about my life, my family, the Peace Corps—everything rippled through me as if the mysteries of life were an open book. I felt clarity as never before. I felt so grateful to be able to experience and perhaps integrate whatever special virtue any particular culture offered. Each had its own jewel. In the midst of my revelation, I felt someone close by. A tiny shepherd girl shyly approached. My heart opened with unconditional love. She stood there and smiled back. I felt her heart. Without speaking, we communicated very deeply.

From there, my perceptions continued to open, and I welcomed but feared the changes. My adventures continued, and often I defied my limitations by pushing myself to keep up with others. One day, my denial caught up to me, and I suffered a major fall that ripped the tendons and ligaments in my impaired knee, and my life as world-explorer came abruptly to a halt. This crisis officially began my healing journey, but it got worse before it got better.

Reluctantly, I returned to the states for rehabilitation, but didn't complete the course. The exercises were boring, I hated being in the US—too fast, too materialistic, too crazy. I flew to Scotland. I had read about the Findhorn Foundation, a community that practiced natural living and alternative therapies. The atrophy of my leg muscles and my chronic curvature caused sciatica of my left hip. I listened to those lectures on self-healing, and I committed myself to the process. My pain served as a wonderful motivator. I received my first massage and was pain-free for four days! Massage became an integral part of my life.

I was invited to London to take a weekend workshop in "rebirthing," which releases mental and emotional tension through practicing certain breathing patterns. The workshop leader inspired me—his own healing journey involved many physical problems, and he was so full of love. He became my mentor. He recognized me as a healer, and suggested that I return to the United States to address my chronic problems.

I chose California, because I wanted to study with Elizabeth Kübler Ross, which I did. I returned to work in the hospital. It had been well over five years since my experience and I was nervous. When I walked in, however, I was blessed with a vision. I saw all of the energy fields of these premature babies in a high-paced thirty bed unit. I was literally struck by a delicate, sweet, Divine presence. I experienced their vulnerability and the purity of their essence, amidst the tension of the working medical personnel. I saw myself years ago, taking care of infants, and being so involved in the technology that I lost sight of their sensitive beings. That changed.

When it was possible to hold them, I would place them on my chest and breathe with them, heart to heart. Our breathing would entrain, and the connection felt like pure love. They would relax, and hopefully feel safe. When they were too sick to hold, I would place my hands on their backs or abdomens and send them energy. At the same time, I would tell them where they were and why. I would explain to them that their parents had not abandoned them, and that they were healing. At times, I would say affirmations. I encouraged mothers to visualize themselves holding their infants on a regular basis, so that at least energetically they could bond with and love their babies.

Personally, I was devoted to my own healing. Chiropractics and Rolfing totally shifted my framework. Weekly breathing sessions deepened my insight to my past. The pain and darkness

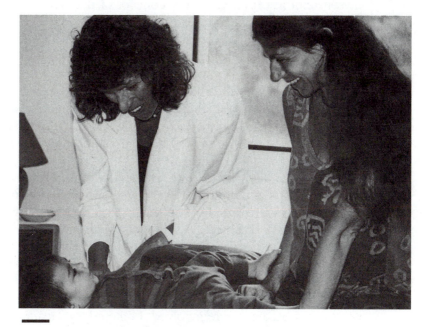

Photograph courtesy of Elaine Criscione

emerged to be healed. As I moved through it, my energy increased and my physical pain decreased. I studied movement. I became more graceful. I took dance classes that awakened my inner beauty.

I corresponded with my mentor on a regular basis. Eventually he invited me back to work with him in Europe. We worked together full-time for one year. He pushed me into process on a continuous basis. I learned energy work from him. I watched him teach groups. He encouraged me to start teaching, so tentatively, I began to do workshops in massage, movement, and rebirthing. My greatest asset was not a theoretical framework, but rather the depth and insight I had acquired as a result of my own healing.

It was my mentor who introduced me to the ancient Vedic rituals of healing. I lived in two Hindu ashrams off and on for two years. A high priest from India gave me the name *Pujarin*, which means "bearer of the Light." Many core issues surfaced for me there—it was a highly transformative time. My disease process emerged one more time, and this time I could see how to change it. I learned to respond to my own needs, instead of leaving myself until last. I let go of my concept of duty (being a super healer was quite synonymous with the super-nurse syndrome). Unfortunately, though, I was quite ill when I left the ashram. I returned to the home of my mentor. He lovingly supported me through my recovery. I worked in his center for the summer, camping in the vineyards alongside the periphery of his farm. I often sat on the hill overlooking the mountains, especially at night. Being alone and "drinking in the night" was the ritual that grounded my spirit into my body. I prayed for guidance for my next step.

My father died and my mother fell ill. My relationship ended, my workshops got canceled for low enrollment. Again, with mixed feelings I returned to the states. I grieved the loss of my European world. I resisted my own roots. My family supported me in the way that they knew and I really appreciated that, but no one was interested in following me in my healing experiences.

Shortly afterwards, in 1986, I joined the American Holistic Nurses' Association. It was still a young, growing organization. Gradually I became more involved. I entered the Healing Touch program in 1991 and became certified as a practitioner and instructor in 1994. I created my own seminar called "Lifedance," which was an eclectic approach to healing through movement and self-care. My target audience has been nurses.

My fervor to heal is still deep in my soul, and the process has been rich. In 1994, I was awarded the wonderful honor of being the American Holistic Nurse of the Year. This is a pivotal event in my life—it is a tangible reminder to me to trust the healing process.

My love for travel continues, and has evolved in focus. I travel extensively nationally to teach workshops in Healing Touch. I have also had the privilege to work as a recovery room nurse with Operation Smile International, a nonprofit organization whose mission is to repair cleft lips and palates of children living in third-world countries. I served with them for two-week stints in both the Philippines and in North Vietnam. I also received sponsorship from the Neonatology Department at Tulane University Hospital, friends and colleagues to travel with Patch Adams on a clown tour to Russia. We visited children in hospitals and orphanages in Moscow and St. Petersburg. My next adventure is to lead a delegation of holistic nurses to India through the People to People Foundation, where we will explore ancient vedic traditions and meet nurses from India.

I am currently still working as a critical care nurse with infants and children. My sense of purpose has strengthened and matured. I continue to offer healing at the bedside. Babies are so pure, and they respond so well to touch. Parents usually respond favorably to my offer. There have been times when I have given Healing Touch treatments to the mothers during moments of crisis. My goal is to see Healing Touch implemented into perinatal situations. The energy work has the potential to enhance bonding, provide safety in the birthing process (emotionally to the baby), and help to optimize the comfort level of the mother during labor, so that she (and the father) can be focused on receiving and welcoming their sacred creation. An additional benefit is for the baby to receive Healing Touch right after birth, for accelerated recovery, and of course, to preserve the innate ability to connect to sacred or therapeutic presence.

The challenge that remains in the hospital is being able to sustain a therapeutic presence throughout the high pace, the tension, the pain, and the crises. What sustains healers is the idea that there is an intrinsic order to the disease/healing process. It is not simply pathology crying out for cure. It is consciousness preparing itself for the opportunity of change, growth, and transformation. Those of us who have experienced the process serve as role models for those who seek to do the same. We expand our concepts beyond the physical into a sacred perspective that can serve as a grounding cord for both the patient/client and/or family.

In 1988, I contributed an excerpt to Charlotte McGuire's *Visions of Nursing*. I visioned nursing students doing "their personal work" to heal. Once they understand their pain, they can be with others in theirs. The resulting commitment and growth creates the role of healer within the nursing framework. It is a role of dignity, compassion, and love. Our own healing as individuals will heal the collective and revolutionize our health care system and the world.

It is time.

LONG-TERM
CARE NURSES

6

INTRODUCTION

The population of the United States and many other nations is aging. The age group of the old, old, persons over 85 years of age, is the fastest growing segment of elders. As such, chronic care needs are on the rise and agencies designed to care for persons with these complex needs are increasing. Many nurses begin their schooling in acute care settings with an occasional rotation to a long term unit. A few committed souls choose to return to those settings following graduation. The nurses profiled in this section chose the path of healing with long term care needs.

As you read their stories, think if you would like these nurses to care for you or your family. Consider these nurses' skills in interpersonal relations and how they developed these skills largely through their own wounding and recovery process. It is this process that has made them stronger and contributed to the process that made them healers.

Rita Benor
RGN, RM, RNT, RHV, Cert. Ed. Couns. Cert., M. BAFATT

Psychotherapist, Autogenic Training Therapist, Bach Flower Practitioner, Lecturer in Complementary Therapies/Medicine, Bishopsteignton, Rockville, Maryland

Throughout my life providence has brought me many lessons about healing. These lessons have shown me my own woundness and how healing may come in many forms: through medical science, in the compassionate skilled touch of a nurse or friends, and through the subtle potency of psychotherapy or homeopathy. The method and vehicle may differ, but all are healing. What matters is the willingness of the individual to become whole and of those around the person to open themselves to the mysteries of healing which brings about this *wholing*.

I have lived all of my life in England. Through many generations my family has possessed gifts of healing through the laying on of hands. It was commonplace for me to observe family, friends, and neighbors receiving healing, so as a child I grew up feeling comfortable with the notion of helping to heal in a relaxed and communal way. However, I was to become the first to express an interest in taking these qualities and interests into professional clinical settings in becoming a nurse.

Between the ages of four and ten I suffered frequent, debilitating throat and ear infections. I was well attended by our family physician. On reflection, I realize how holistic his compassionate and caring approach was. In caring for me he was constantly mindful of my family and of my mother's vulnerability in becoming a widow when I was only four; of the recurring patterns of illness and diseases in the family, of bronchitis and the loneliness of my wartime widowed aunt left to raise young children. He never failed to look beyond the presenting symptoms. He showed a balanced approach in helping. Thoughtfully appreciating the established coping skills within the extended family who were rebuilding their lives and adapting to losses in post-war Britain, he never failed to ask each one of us how we were doing. I know that this loving, caring physician instilled in me a desire to value and recognize medical sciences and at the same time to respect the fragility and strengths of human nature and how we can be instrumental in helping nature to heal others. It is the personal investment of the caregiver underpinning the medical technology who brings about the deeper processes of healing. Dr. Smith set aside the science and acknowledged the strengths and fragilities of human nature and how strong and resourceful the nature of being human can be when held with love and respect.

My experiences with the medical and nursing professions were further enhanced when I was ten years old. I was hospitalized for nearly a month when I had a tonsillectomy complicated by a severe bout of mumps. I had had very little contact with nurses until this admission. I found the penicillin injections so very painful and was alone and afraid, and I desperately missed my family. I began to see and experience the differences in the nurses. Some, despite their smile, did not extend themselves beyond their task. Others listened, talked, and played with us children. Although play therapy is now commonplace, it was virtually unknown in the 1950s. I noticed how much other children in the ward responded to the efforts of those nurses who extended a caring relationship.

At the age of thirteen I identified three potential career routes. I wanted to be a nurse, a teacher, and a researcher. Like all young people I knew that it was not possible to achieve everything at the same time. Now, halfway through my fourth decade, I realize I have achieved all three, and more. I have also been able to hone and to share my innate talents and gifts within the mystery of healing through clinical applications of well-developed intuitive abilities.

My initiation into nursing was mixed. I entered nursing school very idealistic. I was disappointed to see how unfeeling and soulless some of the experiences of caring for ill and dying people were made to be in the hospital setting. I became disillusioned and left after only six months. I worked as a secretary within a psychiatric hospital with direct contact with patients. My idealism changed to seeing the constraints on a national health system that had the desire to care and feel compassion but was constrained by limited financial and human resources.

My confidence and determination resurfaced and I reentered nursing with a more tolerant and accepting attitude and went on to thoroughly ground myself in the art and science of nursing. I found the work physically and intellectually challenging and enjoyed the companionship of other men and women seeking to change the face of illness.

Nurse training in the mid 1960s was still strongly influenced by the dominant medical model with its reductionistic approaches. It was to be more than a decade before British nursing gained professional confidence and independence, following the example of nursing models so favorably growing in the United States.

Throughout my nursing, I was convinced that more could be done for those distressed through illness or disease. I considered my training at the time to be a fulfilling and exciting experience, but at the same time I felt something lacking in the environment that reduced individuals to working parts that had to be put right. This was a system that also did not value and honor the individualism of the nurse.

My journey began as I qualified as a registered nurse and as a staff nurse in gynecology and enjoyed working with women's health. I moved on to training as a midwife. This led to a wider experience and understanding of life, from the miracle of its beginnings to the challenges of its ending in deaths of stillborn children and of the bereavement of families. It became clearer and clearer to me that nursing was not about curing problems but about helping people to deal with life. While not minimizing illness, I began to appreciate that the current climate of health care focused too much on the disease and too little on the healthy aspects of the individual. What followed was twelve years of developing my professional expertise, working within various hospital environments and then broadening my appreciation of the impact of health and illness across the ages by working as a community nurse and health visitor. My clinical work grew and I was better equipped to identify the missing link in hospital-based practice. I saw how hospitalizations marginalized people from their community. I began to see the healing role of the nurse in helping to integrate the experience of illness, to empower patients to come into their wholeness. I saw so many lessons from illnesses which traditional caring frameworks did not address. The innate healer within me was surfacing to explore these deeper issues in healing. There were few who shared my awareness. My intuition told me to wait and be patient, that soon there would be others awakening to these awarenesses. I was drawn to meditate for self-nurturance as I waited for these new frontiers to develop. This also led me to awareness of a need to address the parts of myself that were broken and unwhole.

My interest in psychology led me to train in counseling. My career embraced many of my talents and skills, and I became amoungst the first nurses in the UK to work as a bereavement counselor, genetic counselor, and researcher within an obstetric unit. Being alongside a woman and her partner at a time of loss, whether it be a still birth, or a baby with severe abnormalities, is a demanding and privileged experience. By this time I had suffered my own losses. I had miscarried my first child and knew the feeling of painful disappointment. My loss deepened my empathy. I was moved at the strength of mothers and fathers and shared many tremendously moving moments. One such time was the experience of being with a young mother who was pregnant with twins. She went into premature labor at just twenty-two weeks when her husband was out of town. Her first baby, so tiny, was born just alive. Her second was stillborn. As I sat with her the stillness was such that I had never felt before. She sat on her bed holding the dead baby. I sat next to her in a chair, holding the soon-to-die firstborn baby. We spoke very little. There was a peace and connection that was beyond words, between two people who had not even met before. During the following two hours we passed the babies to each other, taking it in turn to hold them. I stayed with her until her husband arrived and shared with them the grief of their losses.

Lasting and penetrating energies of those moments have stayed with me. When I reflected then, as now, on what took place, I recalled the sacredness of being open, without judgment, to a natural event. In those sharing moments many things had been taking place, simple but effective healing gestures. I was moved to hold and touch in a loving way, feeling the gentleness of the baby as it breathed softly without struggling, letting both of our tears flow and through a generosity of spirit accepting that even in the light of such a loss nature had provided an opportunity for a letting go into bereavement, and from there into a deeper awareness towards healing.

My work also brought me to explore in a wider context the effects of these human tragedies on the midwives and doctors. For the most part they had been excluded from the deeper healing which I was called upon to facilitate. I came to realize that I could enhance the healing benefits by involving and not isolating staff. I set up experiential workshops exploring healing around bereavement, encouraging the staff to identify with their own needs and to develop a fuller connectedness with their patients.

I studied and then became a teacher of Autogenic Training (AT), a profound form of relaxation that addresses physical, emotional, and spiritual aspects of life. Both my own practice of AT and my experience of teaching AT to others enhanced my understanding of the mind-body connection. I extended my repertoire to include visualization, creative writing, drawing, Therapeutic Touch, and Bach flower remedies. I am also indebted to my husband, Dr. Dan Benor, for helping me to talk and publish about the deeper issues in the healing process which before I had been rather hesitant to share. Touch has been an enormously potent intervention that TT helped me to develop.

Life is too short to master all of the many ways of healing. I often refer my clients to homeopaths, osteopaths, aromatherapists, Alexander teachers, and other psychotherapists and complementary therapists who can add dimensions of healing to the therapeutic challenges brought by patients. Healing is a community experience. Having explored these modalities for myself and my patients, I went on to teach and lead experiential workshops internationally to introduce other caregivers to these approaches.

At all time I respect and value traditional science. Complementary healing modalities should never be used to avoid or bypass conventional medical practice. I am opposed to setting up competition that may disadvantage the patient. Terminology like "alternative" should be avoided if an integrative approach is to be developed.

While change is possible, it cannot occur overnight. I have met opposition. Conflicts of interest can be stimulated if traditional practitioners feel threatened when making changes to the usual ways of practice. As a nurse healer I learned to be patient and tolerant, while not compromising what I know to be true, potent, and right within the whole person care. I keep my heart grounded with the help of my head, which has been educated in scientific skepticism, grounded in research. I have been encouraged and helped by the observations of other pioneers in the humanization of caring.

I have been committed to building bridges, and to that end, founded The British Holistic Nurses' Association in 1992. To make time to do this work, as well as to share my approaches to the whole person through lecturing, leading workshops, and writing, I found I had to leave my work in the National Health Service in order to prevent overload and burnout. I now work independently as a consultant nurse lecturer in complementary therapies and holism. This is parallel to my work as a psychotherapist and AT therapist. I will soon undertake training as a homeopath.

My personal growth and healing continue, not only through my professional work but also through my lessons in being a wife and mother, as well as in my enjoyments of cooking, quilting/patchwork, growing herbs, and meeting with kindred spirits.

I feel enormous pride in being grounded in my first love—nursing, and have greatly valued my scientific background. This has been instrumental in adding to my understanding of the subtleties of the mind-body connection. I have discovered the complexities of what it means to be human. In my own healing journey I have greatly appreciated so many wonderful teachers and healers. In finding my own woundedness, I have learned to understand so much about the meaning of healing. I have met with opposition when talking about subtle energy medicine, such as TT, homeopathy, and even psychotherapy, but have realized that nothing is gained by taking these as a personal rejection or criticism. It is important to honor the established way of reasoning. I believe we should talk, write, and research about healing and how instrumental nursing can be in order to help those who are just starting their journeys along these paths. Many are afraid of challenging the system which is resistant to change. Many have to be diplomatic in order to relate with their place of employment. At the same time, we must do our best not to be compromised into not honoring what we have found to be true and helpful. We must realize that it is only a matter of time before attitudes will change. I openly speak about my belief that no single healing modality is the answer. Human nature is complex. Just as there are many ways of feeling, thinking, and being, so too are there many ways of working in caring relationships.

Florence Nightingale said the art of nursing was to put patients in the best possible condition for nature to heal them. We must not get bogged down in methodologies and forget that it is the person that makes the decisions at soul level for her or his own life. I was taught that illness was something to be suffered and cured, without a great deal of thought about why the illness occurred, why now, or what can be learned from the experience. We must remember not to get in the way for nature to take over.

Wailua Brandman
RN, MSN, CS, NP

Instructor of Nursing, Advanced Practice Program, University of Hawaii at Manoa, Manoa, Hawaii

I was born in Indianapolis, Indiana. My parents were both raised in rural Indiana, and attended the same high school. My father was descended from the English Talkingtons (maternal) and a refugee from the Bolshevik Revolution of 1917 (paternally); my mother descended from Mayflower stock (maternal) and the presidential Harrisons. As I grew up, my family lived in Illinois, Iowa, Oklahoma, Tennessee, and Texas, exposing me to variations in culture and climate. In junior high school, my class took a field trip to the Iowa State School and Hospital, and I witnessed a wide range of mental illness and retardation. I was most powerfully influenced by my exposure to a 22-year-old man who was severely mentally retarded. This man was diapered and drooling, laying in a large crib, unable to speak or attend to his own needs. Seeing him there evoked the most profound experience of caring I ever had. I decided on that day to help, in whatever way I could, people who were helpless and dependent. Throughout high school I felt that I wanted to be a physician, although this was influenced largely by my father's drive for capital gain melded with my own desire to help the infirm heal. Before entering college at the University of Oklahoma, I worked at an emergency room, on my mother's counsel, to validate my intention to major in pre-med. It was there, at the age of 17, that I first witnessed the performance of doctors and nurses ministering to the infirm. It became clear to me that the physician role could not satisfy my life's ambition, that the nurse was the one whose caring most closely matched mine. I applied to the next class at the nursing school affiliated with that hospital, and was rejected. I was told that I was an "underachiever," and that I should just go ahead and apply for medical school.

My first two years in college were not satisfying, as I changed my major back and forth from pre-med to psychology to journalism. I ended up transferring to a smaller school, and continued the academic dance, majoring in pre-nursing (which was non-existant at the time), then psychology, then back to pre-nursing. I dropped out of college one semester before graduation because I was disillusioned with the caliber of the faculty and still unsure of my direction. There seemed to be no clarity in what I was doing there. At the age of 23, I watched an acquaintance of mine become an RN through an associate degree program in Dallas. That inspired me to enter the AD program, where I began to excel academically and politically in the nursing arena. Nursing school also marked my first foray into theater acting, which I enjoyed immensely, and I continued to be active in the theater for fifteen years on stage and screen. Fresh out of nursing school, I took a job recovering Dr. Denton A. Cooley's open heart patients in Houston. I was profoundly aware of the post-cardiotomy, transient psychoses these patients experienced and began to study dream analysis and symbolism at the Carl Jung Education Center in Houston. Of course, personal analysis went hand in hand with the course work.

Within six months, an opportunity presented itself to move to New York City. With much excitement, I relocated and took a position at Bellevue Psychiatric Hospital on a treatment and research unit that was run by New York University. I also continued my personal analysis with an analyst who was a protegé of Carl Jung.

I completed my BS in Special Studies in Psychology. This period was extremely frustrating for me, and taught me much about my personal anger. I was very naive about bureaucracy, and very idealistic about patient care. I had carefully formulated creative programs designed to reintegrate the psychotic patient, but was continually told by administration, "No. You can't do that." I finally managed to start some programs that had never been attempted before at Bellevue, like a patient newspaper.

In New York City I experienced many cultures and learned that life's goal is to enjoy life and live love. Besides working as a nurse, I sang and danced off-Broadway, modeled, had my own catering business, avidly studied about the holographic paradigm, and free-lanced as a word processor, learning well that another key to happiness is being a well-rounded person. After three and a half years of inpatient psychiatric nursing, I decided to enroll in a post-graduate psychotherapy training program in Manhattan, and began doing outpatient psychotherapy, which I continued in private practice after completion of the training.

In 1979, I married Ann Forman, who recognized and awakened even more the healer within myself. She also introduced me to the Sufi Order of the West, a universal spiritual movement that embraces the spiritual experience of all religions, known and unknown. There were numerous other teachers of the spiritual realm, and I was eager to see and to hear all they had to offer.

Later, while pursuing the Master of Science in Nursing degree at Yale University, I participated as staff in the first and second Annual Love and Health Congress at Southern Connecticut State University in New Haven. These two annual gatherings of people had a great impact on me, and gave further consensual validation to my work as a nurse healer. Also while at Yale, I had the great fortune to know Virginia Henderson, who is often called the Florence Nightingale of American Nursing. She inspired me to always carry with me and share the essence of nursing as the two of us perceived it—unconditional love.

Another nurse, Joanne Marchione, once wrote that the role of the nurse would one day be that of consciousness counselor, and that is what my practice as a nurse healer is all about. I identify a patient/client's life pattern while in relationship to him/her, then I assist that person to acknowledge the pattern as it is without judgment. This awareness by the patient/client of his/her pattern is enough to begin the healing process. All this is done with the use of language, symbols, emotions, intellect, intuition, knowledge of the physical reality, and an underlying essence of unconditional love. As a psychiatric/mental health nurse practitioner, and consultation liaison clinical nurse specialist, I work part-time in an emergency room, and part-time in an employee health setting where I see essentially well people and urgent care patients. I have just recently become an instructor of nursing at the University of Hawaii at Manoa. My goal is to create a primary care role for a mental health population in Hawaii, where there has never been a role for this type of nursing.

One of the biggest challenges I have had to meet has been the hypersensitivity of traditionalists to nursing's evolution into the domain of consciousness and energy. Intuitively, most nurses are aware of this realm; however, I have found that it is often more productive to show others how it works before trying to explain it or teach them about it. One's sensitivity to language can often be a deterrent to forward movement.

In Hawaiian, the word "Wailua" means two fresh waters (or rivers) coming together in one vessel, forming a fountain spraying water and light, going into the darkness; nurturing, supporting, flowing; figuratively, it means the paradox in one. My message to others who would be healers is to know yourself well, the light and the dark; explore the connection of all life—conscious light, learn about the transpersonal caring moment, as formulated by Jean Watson, and live unconditional love in your life as much as you are able.

Susan B. Collins
RN, MS, FNP, HNC

*Clinical Director, North Country
Community Health Center,
Flagstaff, Arizona*

I was born on Columbus Day in 1938
in Mineola, New York, to Bess and Bill
Ballantyne, and except for being late to
the birth, life was pleasant and relatively
uneventful.

As a firstborn, who was supposed to be a
boy but turned out to be a girl, I reveled in all things boyish.
Guns, cowboys and Indians, war, and dirt lots that turned into fox-
holes were my playground. As I grew older I wanted to be a doctor and operate on people.

My brother, three years younger, was my shadow and we
had neighborhood gangs and I was the leader. In those days the
gangs were age 8 through 11 and rode bicycles and shot cap pis-
tols at each other.

As time passed and adolescence moved into full swing I discovered boys as other than pals and giving in to hormonal urges
found girl clothes, lipstick, and the boy on the next block. Career
decisions in my day were simple; girls were either teachers, sec-
retaries, or nurses. I listened to the "wisdom" of my parents and
went to nursing school. Besides, I never did well in Latin class and
you needed Latin to be a doctor.

After graduation I found myself in the OR as an RN scrub
nurse and occasionally got to sew parts of someone together.
Three years of being entranced with the highly technical skills of
the OR ended as I felt that something was missing. I took up
teaching nursing and moved out to the units and worked with
patients who were awake.

I still thought about possibly going to medical school but
marriage and family intervened. I still listened to my parents and
did what was expected of me.

My oldest son was born not breathing, and after a long
resuscitation was alive but over the next few years clearly had

brain damage, fairly severe with seizures, and cerebral palsy that kept him from walking and talking and other things.

Until that time I had this personal glass bubble that shielded me from the hurts of the world. This occurrence clearly broke my bubble and left me feeling very vulnerable, something that was to be a turning point in my healing journey.

I sought to heal my wounds with knowledge of the handicapped child. I displaced my anger at the unjustness of it all by focusing on organizations that fought for schooling and services for brain damaged children of all ends of the spectrum.

I had another son who was birthed by cesarean section thereby saving us from one more handicapped child. We found the Doman Delacato method of patterning and retraining of neurological pathways and spent three intense years trying to "cure" Mark and make him normal. The gift I found from this was learning to ask others for help. I had to come to the end of my personal rope and abilities and learn to swallow my pride and ask others to do for my son. It was a difficult but also a rewarding experience and learning. I discovered community, sharing, giving and receiving, and the gift of receiving that we can give to others.

I found my spiritual connection through this time and internalized my feeling of self-worth and self-love, on the "no matter what or who" level. I found the strength to end a marriage that was not right and begin a partnership that was.

Through this I spent much of my time with others in a helping, caring mode. When I was younger it was motivated out of my

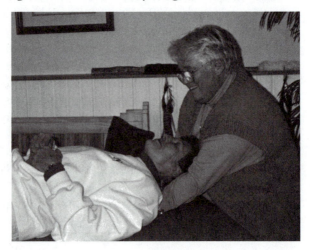

need to be with someone else or feel less than or not wanted. After my internal awakening I spent time alone in peace and harmony with myself and spent time with others in a new way—a way of sharing and not expecting something in return.

Somewhere in my late thirties I discovered the concept of reincarnation and found the thought so freeing. I could cast aside my fears of not "doing it right" and concentrate just on the doing. If I didn't get "it" right this time, oh well, there would be another until I "got it."

As I restudied nursing theorists during my later years, I became happy and proud to be a nurse. I could cast off the need to be a "doctor" and enjoy what I had indeed become. Nursing has a special place with people that is truly sacred. In my younger years I couldn't see that and now I can.

I "discovered" holism and seeing the whole person, natural therapies, and energy. Being with people now is a sacred trust and I enjoy every moment of it. Along the way I became a family nurse practitioner and my patients call me "doctor" because I am their primary health care provider. I correct them and say I am a nurse and proud to be one.

My patients or clients, whichever setting you wish, have often told me of healing moments where I played a part or how my being there influenced their healing process. I choose to see myself as an instrument or agent of a power far greater than myself. I come to the interaction without expectations and with the knowledge that whatever is the highest good for the person I am interacting with at that time will come forth. This approach keeps my ego from getting in the way. I often surprise myself at some of the words and "wisdom" that comes out of my mouth and yet it seems to be just what the person needs to hear. My guiding principal is that each person I interact with is a family member, "mother, father, sister, brother," and I treat them as I would want my family to be treated. People will respond so differently when they are respected.

I study, learn, and show up for life each day. My son Mark and my mother who recently made the transition continue to teach me about patience, loss, and acceptance of things I cannot change. My grandchildren teach me about the world through a child's eyes and the hope for the future. It all keeps me very busy and basically quite happy. I feel very blessed.

Martha Fortune
RN, MS

Nurse Consultant, Community Nursing Organization, Visiting Nurse Association of New York, New York City, New York

My mother, born on a farm in a snowstorm, was nursed by her mother and "Nanny," my great-grandmother. Two years later, my uncle was born in the hospital and in one month my grandmother was dead of pneumonia. Nanny blamed the poor nursing care. Nanny maintained that her daughter would never have taken ill under her care. The wise woman home care legacy was alive in my family. My life began in Watertown, New York, the third child of six and eldest daughter. I had three imaginary playmates for whom I cared and with whom I shared wondrous experiences. When my brother was hit by a bus he was brought to the hospital dead on arrival. We learned later that the ambulance nurse had resuscitated him, although CPR did not exist. For the two weeks he lay in a coma, my Aunt Regina, an RN, stayed with us. Her knowledge and her ability to take charge were a tremendous support. The seeds of education and nursing know-how were evident here.

As a young woman I loved science. I wanted to apply scientific knowledge to people, preferably in Africa. One day, my dream would come true. At age 16 I worked as a candy striper. The nurses let me observe—and sometimes do—interesting procedures. I went on rounds with my friend (and pediatrician) Dr. Charles Goodnough, who explained the patient's history and queried me for my suggestions. He gave me the gift of expert mentoring, while introducing the idea of a generalist—a romantic, yet very real concept—that has shaped my practice.

One summer, as a nurse's aide in the Emergency Room, I interviewed patients and took vital signs. I reported to the nurse who triaged patients. We performed first aid, and made all initial decisions: how to calm an excited person, to anticipate common problems, and to adjust to different personalities.

My awareness of the healing role began in that one room ER. As most patients were discharged to home after treatment, I observed how crucial a nurturing environment is to healing. By example, each ER nurse taught me to nurture myself and to go with the flow on the job, excellent survival skills. My first nursing job at Massachusetts General Hospital taught me to manage acutely ill patients while rotating shifts, again finding ways to self-nurture. My unit teacher taught me the discipline of identifying one strength and one area to work on every three months. In this way I could monitor my growth and remain balanced in an otherwise hectic, energy-consuming atmosphere. In two years I became the unit teacher, passing along this legacy of intuitive wisdom. I became aware of how non-healing the high-tech workplace was. I moved to Rochester, New York, for some respite offered time out to discern my true vocation. Soon, I applied for and was accepted by Project HOPE. One year later I moved to Tunisia, North Africa, for a two-month tour of duty.

I lived alone and thus made my way in the Franco-Arab world of Carthage and Tunis. I worked six days a week in Charles Nicole Hospital teaching nursing in French to mostly male nurses, whose primary language was Arabic. My powers of observation were heightened. I learned diplomacy. This experience broadened

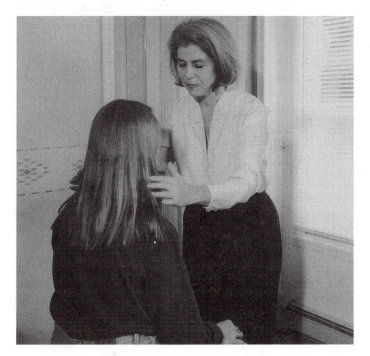

my worldview. Tunisians had few resources, and yet they had a wealth of cultural and ethnic history that carried them through the ravages of illness. I struggled to learn to respect their methods, and to keep an open mind to all practices and beliefs that were helpful to the healing process.

The major hurdle for me was to suspend my Americanized, limited, and righteous approach to health care. As a public health team, we addressed the health care needs of the population while working alongside our Tunisian counterparts.

When I returned to the United States, I obtained an MS in Community Health Nursing, becoming a generalist. I cared for individuals and families in the context of community. Working in people's homes I saw firsthand the importance of not just healing the wound, but of supporting the friends and family in their treatment of the patient as well. As a public health nurse, I lobbied for third-party reimbursement for nurses. I envisioned a return to neighborhood nursing, and though we got the law passed few nurses, much less prospective patients, have profited from it. The mechanism, however, is in place.

Another obstacle for me was figuring out what I wanted to do. The medical model is insidious in nursing academia. I taught at the university level for six years, and resigned in 1985. Within six weeks I discovered Therapeutic Touch and the world of holistic nursing. I attended many seminars on meditation, yoga, and eastern approaches to healing and psychic development. I embraced this new knowledge; it felt so familiar. This was how I wanted to practice: incorporating the mind, emotions, spirit, and body into the patient's health concept. With my community viewpoint, I felt I had truly come home. The primary challenge: Where could I practice? A position at a neighborhood health center launched my holistic practice. I offered continuing education classes in Therapeutic Touch. I worked as a private duty home hospice nurse where I had the opportunity to incorporate TT, reflexology, massage, and guided imagery. Each new modality was introduced into my practice. I charted my interventions, along with any responses, and explained them to my fellow nurses if they asked. Soon I began to feel that nurses needed healing. Many had become disenfranchised from their true desire to help others, and the medical model dissipated their natural healing qualities. The holistic nursing concept that I read about spelled out in detail what

I already knew in my heart: We each have an innate ability to heal ourselves and others. Those of us who continue on this journey are striving to articulate it to others, by our life style, teaching, writing, and practice.

I now work as a hospice nurse at the Visiting Nurse Service of New York. I incorporate this holistic approach to patients from many countries and walks of life. It is healing in the sense of becoming whole, at one with the invisible universal. This has furthered the development of my intuition.

For the past eight years, I have served on the Board of Trustees of the Nurse Healers-Professional Associates, Inc. to support the healing viewpoint in society. During this time, the Board has instituted annual retreats to nurture one another and take a look inward at ourselves and the organization.

My message to those who choose the healing path is first to know yourself, to follow your heart, to do what you love to do, even when you think you cannot, to remain open to the universal energy, and to find ways to nurture, balance, and heal yourself. Stay connected to a group of healers, get regular work on yourself, and find time to be alone. Play. In the great example of my teacher Dora Kunz, laugh.

Susan Luck
RN, MA

HIV Patient Coordinator, Health Educator, Stratogen Health of Miami Beach, Miami Beach, Florida

My impulse to be a nurse healer precedes my earliest memories. My father's recollections give me important information into how I chose my life work. My mother became ill when I was very young and I am told that I always wanted to help her and offer comfort. My father recalls the time he came home from work and found me kneeling at her side on the floor after she had fainted. When he entered the living room, he found me beside her on the floor where she had fallen. I was applying a cold compress to her forehead while comforting her with soothing words and massaging her cold hands. My older sister hid in the corner of the room, crying, while I took control of the situation. I had intuitively assessed what was needed and my mother soon regained consciousness. I was not yet four years old at the time. My mother died of metastatic breast cancer just days before my seventh birthday and with a new seven year cycle beginning, I believe I was initiated into the special world of the wounded healer.

As a teenager, I looked forward to visiting my ailing grandmother in a nursing home because I wanted to help the elderly who appeared so alone. We would write letters to their grandchildren; I would comb the long gray hair of the old women with toothless smiles and kind, sad eyes. I was touched by their spirits. I continued on to be a candy striper until I entered college and studied nursing.

In the 1960s, being raised in a family that valued hard work and independence, there was never a question in my mind of my professional direction. Nursing was always challenging to me, although not in the intellectual sense. The intellectual side of me excelled throughout my studies. It was my intuitive side that was finely tuned and that got me into the most trouble! I was often admonished for staying with a patient for too long; or for holding their hand, or sitting on the bed and breaking sterile technique. I was told that my behavior was "unprofessional" because I cried when a patient that I had been caring for died. Even worse was when I shared my tears with the patient's family. When I graduated from school and became a registered nurse at eighteen, I began the adventure of exploring my nursing career and my potential to become a nurse healer.

My curiosity and love for people led me to the world of the mind—a thread that would weave a colorful tapestry over the years. Psychiatric nursing in those days relied on personal interaction rather than on medications. I worked in psychiatric units, drug treatment facilities, and alcoholism programs. I loved listening to people tell their stories. I was fascinated by the diversity and the sameness of the human condition. I took advanced courses in psychology and eventually studied psychosynthesis, learning imagery through a psychospiritual perspective. My search to see where I could "fit" into the system as a nurse continued over the next decade.

In the mid 1970s, I migrated to California where an early awareness of holism was already emerging. I became a head nurse in a hospital-based alcoholism treatment program. The program was known as a CARE unit. The acronym stood for: Comprehensive Alcoholic Rehabilitation Environment. This was Berkeley, 1975.

I was encouraged to hug my patients, dim the lights, and play soft music so to temper the effect of the DTs when they were withdrawing from multiple substances. The philosophy of this program fit me like a glove. Although standing orders for medications were always available, the challenge was to gently guide these individuals through their process creatively and holistically. Nobody had a seizure on my shift! I became interested in yoga and nutrition during this period while working on my personal health issues. I began to bring yoga and relaxation techniques on to the unit. The connection between the mind and the body was not yet understood in this culture, but my curiosity and intuition led me on. I needed to understand the uniqueness and diversity of humankind.

I began my studies in anthropology at the University of California in 1976. After studying for three months, I volunteered to be part of an emergency team to go to an isolated region in the highlands of Guatemala to administer emergency health care following a major earthquake. I was to integrate it into my field study component. I was supposed to stay for six weeks; I stayed over one year. My own life and consciousness was uprooted by my contact with the community of Maya from the moment I arrived. The earthquake occurred at three a. m. and as the mountains trembled, the terra cotta tiled roofs tumbled and buried all beneath. The final count numbered ten thousand. I arrived in this moment of chaos and confusion, vulnerability and despair. I was not prepared for the world that unfolded nor the gift of the privilege of being part of this dramatic cultural event.

After the immediate emergency care was administered, the villagers that came to the "mash" unit and field hospital presented symptoms that we were ill equipped to understand as western-trained practitioners. Women brought themselves and their children, often diagnosing themselves with "Susto." I never learned that illness category in my nursing training! The symptoms included loss of appetite, abdominal problems, depression, and fevers. Western diagnosis and treatments did not offer relief. ("Susto" comes from the verb, "asustar," which means "to frighten" in Spanish.) One day, a woman I had befriended in the village came to the clinic and told me that she was six months pregnant and had experienced Susto during the earthquake when her house caved in and several family members died. She said she would not have a healthy baby and asked what she should do. Accompanied by her local midwife, I asked her midwife what she thought. She told me that she wanted Lilian to go and consult with the shaman because only the shaman could cure the Susto by contacting her ancestral spirits that dwell in the mountain caves. Lilian then told me her story of how the fright of the earthquake and the sadness of her loss had affected her unborn child. I offered to accompany the woman to the local healer. This became my introduction and initiation into the larger cosmology of healing and the many levels of health and illness; body, mind and spirit.

This moment introduced me to so many questions and possibilities into the realms of healing. This experience inspired my own search leading me on the path to ask the questions in the years to follow, "What is health?", "What is Healing?" As I studied with the local shamans over the next year, I also worked with the local women, who were eager to gain more control over their own lives and insure the continuation of the health of their children. In highland Guatemala, one out of five children dies before the age of five. Poor sanitation, contaminated water, and malnutrition are endemic. I began nutrition classes and community gardens. The women wanted to learn new tools for health and survival for their children, community, and culture. It was ironic that I would have to re-educate them as to the value of corn and black beans, the staple of their diet. Many had drifted into the world of sugar, white bread, and coca cola. Much of this had to do with losing their ancestral lands to large landowners, and to the cutting down of trees for firewood, and the eventual erosion of the soil.

As the community began to organize, local leaders began to mysteriously disappear. Taking control of one's life, if you are a Mayan Indian, was seen as subversive by the powers that governed with an iron fist. One night the military arrived, and in the morning many people had disappeared. Over the course of the next several years, tens of thousands of indigenous people would be massacred and thousands more would flee into the mountains and find their way over the northern border into the jungles of southern Mexico. I was the only foreigner that remained in the community, and the town elders told me my life was in danger. I left the next day, saying good-bye to my new friends, wondering if I would ever see them again. A decade later, many bodies would be discovered in the clandestine cemeteries that bordered the town.

In 1979, I returned to New York, and became involved in an effort to get information out to the world on the human rights atrocities that were occurring without a voice to tell the story. I became a journalist, and using a pen name, I returned to Guatemala. When that became impossible, I relocated to Chiapas, Mexico, working with the refugees through organizations including Save The Children. I continued working in the areas of nutrition, and self-sufficiency projects including weaving cooperatives and gardens. The cultural survival of the Maya took on a special meaning for me, revealing the struggle of a people and the strength of the human spirit. My work and connectedness to this culture has been a theme in my life in many unexpected ways. I traveled between the two worlds, raising money and awareness while providing health care. During this time, I befriended an indigenous woman, Rigoberta Menchu, who had been brought to New York to tell her story to the United Nations Humans Rights Commission. I offered her my home for shelter and a friendship began that continues today. Rigoberta Menchu went on in her incredible journey to win the Nobel Peace Prize in 1992.

During this time, I continued my studies and in 1980 created my own Bachelors Degree Program in Holistic Health Sciences through the State University of New York, Empire State College. This program became a model for a holistic education curriculum in the years to follow. My interest in Holistic Health came together in Guatemala when I witnessed Susto as a body/mind/spirit model. Psychoneuroimmunology had not yet come into its own, but that was the essence of Susto, a classic PNI model.

I began graduate school in Medical Anthropology at The New School for Social Research in 1981. Of course, my interest was in "Cross Cultural Perspectives in Health and Healing." With Michael Harner as one of my professors, who taught the course on Shamanism, I spent many graduate school hours drumming, chanting, and opening up to the Spirit worlds. At the same time, I was trying to work in the medical model but could no longer endure the institutional mentality. I worked briefly on the Depression Unit of the New York State Psychiatric Institute. I worked the evening shift, but after I brought chamomile tea onto the unit, replacing the customary sleeping pills that kept the patients like zombies, I was informed that I was bringing "untested" drugs into the hospital. I left shortly thereafter.

I began working with a chiropractor specializing in nutritional medicine and began yet another direction of study. I took workshops and read everything I could find. Over time, I developed my own private practice as a holistic nurse, specializing in nutritional counseling. In my search for deepening my own understandings, I took a course in the summer of 1982 at Omega Institute titled "Holistic Health for Health Professionals." There were thirteen people registered for the course, and ten were nurses. I spoke with the director of the Institute and shared my vision that something was going on within the nursing profession that was unique. He suggested that I create a course for nurses, and so I did. For the next several years, I created courses for nurses with titles including "21st Century Nursing" and "The New Nursing." One of the students of the Omega summer program was

Veda Andrus who went on to become the president of the AHNA. As our relationship evolved, we worked on creating a program in Holistic Nursing for the AHNA. I had been carrying the vision to plant seeds in the largest garden possible. Several people worked on the first certificate program. It was launched in 1987 at Clemson University. It was a wonderful moment. That year at Omega Institute, I was awarded the AHNA Holistic Nurse of the Year, an honor that I will always treasure.

As my private practice blossomed, I became involved in developing local holistic nursing programs with two colleagues in New York: Jeanne Ansemo, a holistic nurse for many years and at the time the first nurse president of the New York Biofeedback Society, and Bonnie Schaub, Director of the New York Psychosynthesis Institute. Our shared vision was to touch the core of health and healing for nurses—body, mind, and spirit. We developed a course which is now in its ninth year called "Caring for Ourselves, Caring for Others." As nurses transform their health and gain new awareness, the incredible process unfolds of the nurse healer within. Together we have lectured, written, and participated in international conferences.

The vision of holistic nursing as the healing art that will lead to health care into the twenty-first century, combined with my love of anthropology, led me on a vision mission. For seven years, I worked without funding and with incredible support to produce a documentary for nurses titled "The Heart of Healing: Experiencing Holistic Nursing."

The Aquarius spirit in me saw that this information needed to get out to the largest audience possible as soon as possible. As a new model of health care emerges, and the paradigm shifts, it is essential that nurses emerge as leaders in the twenty-first century. The video* has become a part of nursing education in many schools, used as inservice in hospitals, and shared within the nursing community. Seeds need to be planted and we never know where the wind may carry them. (*See Resource list for Kineholistic Foundation)

My work in nutrition and community health inevitably led me to working with the HIV community. Once again, feeling ahead of my time, I saw holistic health and nutrition as a core component in staying healthy with HIV. Over the years, a few supportive doctors and health centers have allowed me to implement a holistic program for HIV care. After receiving a Ryan White Grant in 1992, I researched and wrote educational materials for both health workers and HIV individuals titled "Staying Healthy with HIV." The books and information have been resource materials for many programs and health centers. The information is still more progressive and relevant than what is available through the standard networks.

In 1993, I moved to Miami in search of a healthier life and I found it. I currently work in a progressive HIV medical center where I have been given the creative task to develop a complimentary health care model for HIV. The center integrates medical care with acupuncture, herbal medicine, nutrition, chiropractic, massage therapy, imagery groups, and a variety of other modalities for mind/body/spirit health. I serve as coordinator of this integrated approach. The HIV community, receptive to the holistic approach, has been a wonderful teacher as I continue to ask the questions about the healing potential. I am beginning to become involved in research and clinical outcomes as another pioneer model demonstrates promise and hope in a medical framework that is limited in both its understandings and approaches.

I have come to appreciate that life is about growth, change, and possibilities. Although one's journey travels in diverse directions, the threads continue to weave the unique tapestry of each one of our lives. I await the next chapter to unfold.

Carol Wells-Federman
RN, MS, MEd, CS

*Co-Director, Chronic Pain Clinic,
Division of Behavioral Medicine,
Beth Israel Deaconess Medical
Center; Associate in Medicine,
Harvard Medical School,
Boston, Massachusetts*

Many healers have influenced my career
as a nurse. Of these, my grandmother had
the greatest impact. I can still see her in my
mind's eye today as clearly as when I was sitting with her over
thirty-five years ago. Short and plump with rosy cheeks and white
hair, she had a gleam in her eye that her wire-rimmed glasses
could not hide. She was not a nurse or a doctor, but she knew
about healing. I remember visiting with her as an eleven year old.
She talked with me as if I was the most interesting person on earth,
and as if there was nowhere else she would rather be, and no one
else she would rather be with. I was not just one of her twenty-
two grandchildren; I was someone she wanted to know. It did not
matter whether I was happy or sad, joyful or hurt, quiet or loud,
she listened to me and guided my growth and understanding.

I had no idea of the gift she was giving me with her respect
and undivided love and attention. Now, after more than twenty
years as a nurse I understand that she was showing me the healing power of presence and relationship—a gift, I would learn, not
so easily passed along.

In 1976, as a naive graduate nurse I thought that helping
people meant curing them. I thought I knew how, so I helped
people physically, mentally, emotionally, and spiritually. I was
unaware that what my grandmother had shown me was essential
to nursing. I discovered, much to my dismay, that I did not know
how to practice both the art and science of my profession. I did
not know how to support healing when I couldn't cure. As a
young, inexperienced nurse working in an acute care, high-tech
environment, I quickly lost any ability to focus holistically.
Prompted by my unconscious need to bolster my own self-esteem

by helping others, I was often overinvolved with patients' needs and unable to maintain clear boundaries. My relationships were based almost entirely upon what I thought others needed and what I could give, not on what I could learn. My oversolicitous helping often overlooked the responsibilities, autonomy, and resources of the people I was trying so desperately to help.

Overwhelmed, I was unaware of how my feelings of uncertainty, disappointment, and frustration affected my body. Constantly holding my breath and carrying increasingly more muscle tension in my neck, shoulders, and low back, I exacerbated an old neck injury to the point where I required long periods of rest and physical therapy. I became increasingly more disenchanted with my career and unable to cope physically and emotionally. After only two and a half years I left acute care nursing.

Interestingly, it was this struggle with physical disability, burnout, and disillusionment that gave me the opportunity to focus my attention on self-care and change. The struggle helped me to slowly recognize what my grandmother had been showing me in developing a healing relationship. Ultimately, the journey led to an understanding that would encourage my return to nursing and continue to guide my practice. It led to the discovery that healing is personal and not something I can give to or get from another. The journey was, and still is, one of growth and of owning the responsibility of taking care of myself, developing healthy relationships, and a balanced life style.

Since my grandmother's death twenty-eight years ago, other gifted teachers, many who are profiled in this book and many who are former patients, have influenced my transition and healing work, some through their writings, others through personal relationship. From Florence Nightingale I came to understand that my responsibility as a nurse was not to cure but to create a healing environment for the patient. Reading her words, "Nature alone cures . . . and what nursing has to do . . . is put the patient in the best possible condition for nature to act upon him," I recognized what my grandmother had been modeling for me all those years ago. This realization significantly influenced my understanding of healing. This perspective allowed me to see that it is the innate capacity of the individual I care for that heals. My responsibility then is to participate in the process with knowledge and compassion.

From Rabbi Harold Kushner, author of *Why Bad Things Happen to Good People*, I learned to redefine success. He helped me realize how much good I can do if I remember that there are things that I can help the patient to heal that I cannot cure. I can support healing by helping patients feel better about what is unfixable. I can help patients heal by letting them know that they are worth worrying about and are good even when they are sick. Kushner tells a story about a little boy whose mother sends him on an errand that takes him much longer than she expects. When the boy returns home his mother says, "Hey, where were you? I was worried about you." He answers, "Oh there was this kid down the street who was crying because his bicycle was broken. I felt bad for him so I stopped to help." The mother says, "You don't know anything about fixing bicycles." "No, of course not," he replies, "I stopped and helped him cry."

This story reminds me that there are always ways to help no matter how impossible the situation may seem, even if it is to help people cry and not leave them to cry alone. For a person who is sick, abandonment is the greatest fear. In a society that does not like to acknowledge pain and suffering and in a health care system that is so technologically sophisticated and organizationally complex, it is a very difficult thing to remember and practice. It is what I could not understand or practice as a young, inexperienced nurse in the ICU.

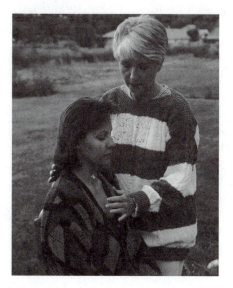

Since leaving acute care, I have had many careers in nursing. I have been a research nurse in epidemiology, a graduate student in health education, a community health educator, a specialist in behavioral medicine, and a graduate and postgraduate educator. During those years, as I was being intellectually influenced by other healers, I was unable to return to clinical nursing until I learned the practice of Therapeutic Touch (TT). It was through this practice and my relationship with the nurses that taught me TT, that I learned to apply the concepts my grandmother, Nightingale, and Kushner had expressed. The ability to be present, to create a healing environment, and to facilitate healing whether or not there is a cure are the essential constructs of TT. The practice necessitates centered attention, focused intention (conscious compassion), and a willingness to "let go" of the outcome. It requires that I understand that I am not using my strength or energy in the process but that I am repatterning or mobilizing the patient's own healing capabilities. Practicing TT has given me a means to be with patients in a compassionate and empathic way while maintaining and encouraging autonomy and growth for both the patient and myself. It has provided many examples of how healing can be facilitated through caregiving. Through this experience I have learned to clarify my responsibility to offer what I can without imposing the outcome and, at the same time, allowing others their contributions. This shift in understanding and practice has helped me to recognize and let go of my tendency to become overinvolved and to better define the boundaries between myself and the patient.

Nine years ago I returned to clinical nursing to work with people who have chronic illness. For the last three years I have been working with individuals who live with daily nonmalignant pain, guiding them in finding ways to cope. Now, from a very different perspective, I am able to witness ordinary people doing extraordinary things. They have shown me the strength of the human spirit in ways I never experienced before. Even with the disability of daily pain, many are able to find inner resources and a capacity to cope that they had not known. They live with the knowledge that their condition may never improve and, in fact, may worsen. Many learn, however, that through their personal efforts, they can develop the kind of life they would want to follow even if their efforts had no impact on the course of their

pain. It is through strengthening the whole, increasing the repertoire of response to and management of stress (chronic pain), and
finding balance within the disequilibrium of pain that they grow,
develop, and provide important lessons for me and others.

They are a constant reminder that healing is never announced
with drums and cymbals, but if I am present and listen, I will hear
healing's subtle but profound sound. I remember a young woman
in the clinic with a very long and complicated history of fibromyal-
sia, abuse, and addiction. She was struggling with many of the
things we were asking her to do for her health and well-being. In
addition, her anger and disappointment with her life was often
directed at us, and this made it exceptionally difficult to stay present with her. She told me one day that her husband wanted her
to go out and buy some new shoes because all her shoes were so
outdated and worn. She, however, saw absolutely no reason to
buy new shoes. I completely missed the message in this statement
until several weeks later when I began to notice that her face was
changing. It was becoming softer; she was wearing a little makeup
for the first time, and coming to clinic with her hair combed. But
I finally heard the subtle sounds of healing when she came in
overjoyed one day to tell me that she had just bought a new pair
of shoes. I had no idea how much she had given up on her future
until she was able to tell me she could now see one for herself.

Finally, from my husband I have learned to cultivate a healthy
sense of humor—essential for a healer. It is very easy for me to forget who is doing the healing. Fortunately, I surround myself with
loving people who help me keep my perspective. Not infrequently
these people are patients with whom I have been working. Just
recently I was interviewing a woman for her discharge evaluation.
She had been suffering for many years with severe crippling
rheumatoid arthritis. We were reviewing how much progress she
had made over the last ten weeks in the clinic, and she was sharing with me how much this had changed her life. I asked her what
she thought had the biggest impact on this change, expecting to
hear that it was something I had taught her in clinic or some sage
statement I had made. She thought for a moment and then said,
quite pleased, "Oh, I was finally able to clean off my desk after 15
years! You can't imagine what this meant to me." Smiling inside
and out, I said, "Actually, I can." My grandmother taught me to listen with my heart, and I am grateful.

Anneke Young,
RN, BSN, CNAT

Director, Wholistic Nursing School at the New Center College, and Associate Director, Wholistic Health Center at the New Center College, Syosset, New York

With healing all around me, it was no surprise that by the time I was seven, I wanted to be a nurse. As a small child, I was surrounded by an interest in healing. My first experiences were with nontraditional healing. My father, a well-known Dutch psychic healer in Rotterdam, the Netherlands, where I grew up, used to practice magnetic healing, a form of laying on of hands. He would place his hands on the area of a person's body that was hurting or diseased, after which the person would inadvertently feel better. My mother also had a strong interest in healing and was often able to take pain away from others. I loved to imitate my dad by putting my hands on the forehead of my mother or brother, trying to alleviate their headaches. I often played doctor and nurse with my dolls, while dreaming about my future as a healer. I pictured myself moving around from patient to patient on a large ward—giving back rubs, adjusting pillows, handing out drinks, and providing comfort to many people.

At the age of seventeen, I started an apprenticeship in a Rotterdam hospital, which at that time was the way students received nursing education. My training involved clinical rotations through every major department of the hospital and allowed for exposure to all of the various specialties. By the time I graduated from nursing school, I had experienced every aspect of nursing and was ready to see the world. Ever since I had visited the United States when I was fifteen, I had been drawn to this country—fascinated with its vastness and convinced that one day I would live in America. One spring afternoon, I finally decided that the time was right to leave my country. I arrived in New York with neither a nursing license nor a driver's license! I moved in temporarily with an uncle, who gave me a bike to get to my first job as a nurse's aid in a local nursing home. Over the next two years, I not only got my driver's license but passed the New York state

Board Examination. I started working in a major medical center on the north shore of Long Island, where I was soon promoted to head nurse at one of the ambulatory dialysis units.

In 1978, a simple act of browsing through the Yellow Pages changed the entire course of my life. While looking for an exercise system I saw an ad for yoga classes being offered at the Institute for Self Development in Manhasset, New York. Several days later at the institute, I met Tina Sohn, a very special woman, who would become my teacher. She and her husband Robert had founded the Wholistic Health Center two years earlier, which was then part of the Institute of Self Development. Today, the Wholistic Health Center, the largest alternative health care facility on the east coast and innovator in wholistic health care, is part of the New Center for Wholistic Health Education & Research, in Syosset, New York.

When I first met Mrs. Sohn and heard about the incredible results she had achieved treating critically ill patients, I was eager to become her student. Tina Sohn is the master and founder of Amma Therapy, a healing art that uniquely synthesizes a Western approach to organ dysfunctions with Oriental medical principles of diagnosis and assessment of the energetic system. As I learned more about Amma Therapy, I realized that this modality is also one of the most logical and practical methodologies of wholistic nursing theory, particularly that of Martha Rogers who has truly influenced my thinking that the energy field is the unifying principle of wholism.

When I asked Mrs. Sohn to accept me as a student she gave me one of my first lessons in wholism—that before I could start helping others, I first had to be healthy myself. She taught me that development of a wholistic practitioner begins with training the physical body. For a wholistic nurse looking to practice Amma as the primary nursing modality, physical strength is absolutely necessary. To be an Amma practitioner, I had to be able to treat my tenth patient of the day with the same attention, sensitivity, and strength as my first. I needed not only strength, but stamina as well. First and most basic, I had to learn the proper techniques for using my hands in palpation and treatment. Through intensive and sometimes strenuous hand exercises, I had to develop the necessary physical strength and sensitivity to the body surface. Hands, I learned, are the wholistic nurse's primary tools.

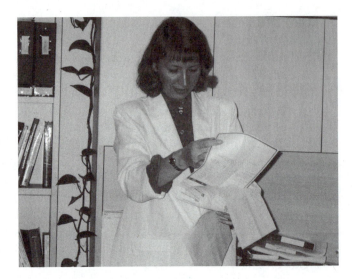

From Mrs. Sohn, I learned about the importance of physical health as a practitioner preparing to treat the ailments of others. I also learned how the training of the physical body produces direct experiential understanding of the body's internal functioning. There is no better way to study living anatomy than by learning to understand one's own organism. I began to study T'ai Chi Chuan to develop this combined academic and experiential knowledge of the human body.

The practice of T'ai Chi Chuan, a Taoist form of exercise and active meditation, helped to increase my level of awareness and to establish control over my own energy system. T'ai Chi Chuan is the effort to create a mind-to-energy-to-physical-body pathway—that is, to establish mind control over the energy so that the energy may properly control and move the body. The mind moves the energy and the energy moves the body. As a result of the concentration and practice of subtle awareness required to master T'ai Chi Chuan, the movement of energy became a cognitive experience for me as a practitioner.

After I started taking lessons in T'ai Chi Chuan and asked Mrs. Sohn if I could start apprenticing, she gave me my second important lesson in wholism—the evolution of a wholistic nursing practitioner also depends on emotional development. Since emotions are part of the bioenergy system and are often responsible for many of the diseases that people experience, we must know the emotional components of disease and understand the way the patient experiences the world. To see and feel another's physical and emotional experiences, great effort must first be made to see and to feel one's own emotional experiences, therefore a fundamental part of becoming a wholistic nurse is the evolution of one's own self-awareness. As I watched Mrs. Sohn, I saw that a true wholistic health professional is one who cultivates concern for the well-being of her/his patients far beyond the normal levels of human concern. This requires that the practitioner first undergo some personal exploration of her/his emotional nature to be able to suspend personal emotions during treatment and give the patient all necessary caring and support. Doing treatment, the physical, psychological, and emotional conditions of the practitioner can directly affect the concomitant areas in the patient, since there can be transmission of energy from the practitioner to the patient. This clearly demonstrates the need for the physical, psychological, and emotional development of the nurse.

The journey of developing as a wholistic nurse under the guidance of Mrs. Sohn was for me a remarkable experience. Being able to help heal others through feeling their inner physical and emotional experience has also helped to develop my own inner being. As I have evolved, I have become more in touch with my spiritual existence and with that of my patients. Once my skills and sensitivity as a wholistic practioner were sufficiently evolved, I began to share what I had learned with other nurses. This led to the foundation of the Pioneer Program in Wholistic Nursing at The New Center, now a 635 clock hour program for registered nurses. The program encompasses all of the components that Mrs. Sohn has taught me over these past years, with subjects and areas taught that are necessary to develop into a true wholistic nurse.

It is through consistent effort to "know thyself" that the nurse uncovers and nurtures the higher potential of human beings, the ability to touch the deeper reality shared with the rest of nature. Through this knowledge and experience, the ability to understand and feel the suffering of others and the comprehension of how to best alleviate that suffering becomes possible. As nurses travel this path of self-discovery and dedication towards helping others, nurses gain not only sensitivity but health, strength, compassion, wisdom, freedom, and joy. They evolve from practitioners to becoming real healers.

Chapter 7

ADMINISTRATIVE NURSES

INTRODUCTION

One usually thinks of an administrative nurse as the person in charge. Indeed, those who serve via the administrative role obtain their position because they are multiskilled: both with academic credentials and clinical work experience. But, you may wonder, how can a nurse both be "in charge" and be "a healer"? Being an administrator is not incongruous with being a nurse healer. Healing is the ability to assist, guide, facilitate, or assist another, or groups of others in the integration of the body, mind, and spirit. Nurses in the administrative role simply work with groups of people rather than with the individual encounters that many practitioners experience. All groups are composed of individuals and those in administration often spend their days with series of individuals via counseling, progress reports, problem solving, and planning patient services.

We hope you read with interest the stories of the following nurses who currently serve in administrative roles. As you read, remember that they, too, were at one time in acute, chronic, education, or independent practice roles.

Jean Sayre-Adams
RN, MA

*Director, Didsbury Trust,
Bath, England*

When I was born on a bleak November day in the panhandle of Nebraska, the mystery of Avalon and ancient magic sang only in my cellular body and in the longing of my soul. I was the granddaughter of pioneers who had made the journey in covered wagons over the Oregon Trail. Their journey had started in England in 1648. They were always pushing ahead to unknown territory. Little did I know that I would be the one that would push so far West as to return to the country of my ancestors in search of what we had known all along. I now live in a magic cottage in England in the midst of Avalon, committed to continuing to reveal those mysteries to myself and others who seek.

Only gradually did I move out of the sandhills of Nebraska, through marriage, to the Colorado Rockies where I first became a nurse, an LVN, out of the necessity to feed five children. In 1969 I made a move to California where I became an RN and went on to get a degree in Holistic Studies. Although it seemed a coincidence that I went into nursing, once I experienced nursing I never imagined doing anything else. It seemed a perfect way for me to become aware of my own struggles, pain, suffering, and eventually start my own healing at the same time being of use to others who were also longing to heal.

It was while working at the University of California at the Cancer Research Institute that I "by accident" attended a class in Therapeutic Touch (TT) taught by Dolores Krieger. TT did not fit into my high-tech nurses training and I put TT on a shelf for the next six months. Then, one night shift when I was desperate to bring pain relief and sleep to a very ill woman, I remembered TT and decided to try it. It worked. I've never looked back.

Within a month I was using TT with most of my cancer patients to help with relaxation and pain relief. Within the next year I had started to use TT in private practice and had joined the staff at the Alternative Therapies Unit at San Francisco General

Hospital as a nurse healer. I used imagery, TT, meditation, and counseling skills with most of my patients/clients. This was in the late 1970s and early 1980s and the largest part of my clientele was a group of people who had strange, unknown symptoms that we now know as HIV/AIDS. That was a time of accelerated growth for all of us and I will be continually grateful for the richness, wisdom and healing I gained from people with whom I worked. I found that the use of TT, imagery, and presence helped my patients relax and deal with pain and to approach their disease with a new awareness. Soon I was asked to begin to show other nurses what I was doing and begin to teach TT in an informal setting.

Independently, or so I thought, I also had the unexplainable desire to travel to the British Isles. I had never before traveled by myself nor traveled outside of the United States except for Canada and Mexico. However, I cashed in some retirement funds, took time out from work, and arrived in Heathrow Airport with six bags. I was going to go backpacking on the Cornish coastlines, and I was, of course, going to meet the Queen. Only the back-packing became a reality, but as one mystical adventure unfolded into another in the southwestern part of England, the Queen faded into the background. One of those experiences led me to give a talk about my work, which at the time was helping to introduce TT into an in-patient setting on an AIDS unit at San Francisco General Hospital, to a group who were attempting a somewhat similar service, the Bristol Cancer Help Center in England. This group went on to become one of the world's first independent cancer help centers. After hearing my talk they then asked me back for the next year, and the next, and the next to talk to them and teach them about TT, imagery, and conscious living/conscious dying.

From 1983 to 1988, I continued to work as a mainstream high-tech nurse in university hospitals in San Francisco and at the same time I continued my private practice and staff work at the Alternative Therapies Unit at San Francisco General Hospital. But during my holiday time, I returned to Great Britain to teach TT and conscious living/conscious dying to interested nurses throughout England, Ireland, Wales, and Scotland.

Becoming aware of the need to participate in the healing of my own wounds before I could be effective in helping others in their healing, I began my personal therapy in 1981. This was a long process and helped me become more sensitive to the pain, struggle, and longing in others. It made me aware of the importance of health care professionals learning to become aware of and breaking out of co-dependent positions. This discovery allows us ways to be with people and come from wholeness rather than need. This, in turn, allows others to discover their own wholeness, and the healing process can start.

Therefore, when some money was offered to me in Great Britain to set up a charity that would address some of these issues, I accepted and a year later moved to England. If I had known what would be required of me over the next five years, I would not have had the courage to do it. Old systems fight hard but they are transforming. Resistance from old systems (National Health Service and religious organizations), promised finances dissolving into the air, the fear from other nurses and managers of any hint of change, and apathy were only a few of the problems I faced.

This charity, the Didsbury Trust, became a registered charity in 1989. It is dedicated to the care, support, and education of nurses and health care professionals through the promotion of the healing arts. Although our role was visioned to be somewhat different in 1989, economics and the changing role of the National Health Service has guided our focus to TT, with the belief that when TT is embraced in its fullest sense, that empowerment and change will occur in those who practice it and in the systems in which they practice. TT is now an accredited course leading to a degree at Manchester University. It is also taught in many university settings in Great Britain. Our goal is to bring the healing arts into mainstream nursing.

As director and administrator of the Didsbury Trust, I spend most of my time teaching classes combining beginning level to degree level in TT and in clinical leadership, change management, conscious living/conscious dying and in the creation of sacred space. As an author, I write books and am on editorial boards of nursing journals. I also participate in conferences and committees focusing on the healing of self and others, and speak on radio and TV programs that are concerned with health and healing. I also commune with all life forms that pass through my isolated magic cottage.

Every day I learn something new. Messages I would have for others who want to follow the path of healing and of the heart would be as follows:

- Know, love, and stay true to yourself.
- Learn to express yourself to others as clearly and accurately as possible in the moment.
- Trust in the universe and stay strong.
- Be open to anything and everything.
- Live and love as fully and as consciously as possible in the present moment.
- Enjoy the dance.

Ernestina Handy Briones
RN, PhD

Nursing Administrator, Valley Baptist Medical Center, Harlingen, Texas

I was born and raised in Pharr, Texas, 15 miles north of the Texas/Mexican border and 250 miles south of San Antonio, Texas. I am one of four children born to Alvina Garcia and William Henry Handy. I am of Mexican and German descent. Both of my parents' families were affected by wars.

My mother, Alvina Garcia, was born in Hidalgo, Texas, but raised in Mexico. During World War I, my grandfather decided not to fight for the United States and returned to Reynosa, Mexico, to raise seven orphaned children. My mother became a Spanish teacher and public speaker. During World War I, my paternal grandfather escaped to South Texas from Michigan when the U. S. government was placing Germans in camps in Michigan. Thomas Handy married Lucia Moreno and came to own about 200 acres next to the Schuster Farms. My father, William, was one of sixteen children. He, like the rest of his siblings, were illiterate and grew up raising farm animals. I currently own the Handy cemetery.

I decided to become a nurse when I was thirteen years of age and spent the summer caring for a six-year-old cousin with whooping cough. Manuel, my cousin, was also minimally physically handicapped. I became a nurse because I wanted to take care of the sick. An influencing factor was the hospital building. It represented a job inside a secure building that would not be affected by the weather such as rain or hurricanes. The hospital symbolized a clean environment with air conditioning, good lighting, and a check every two weeks. Working in the cotton fields during the summer and growing vegetables during weekends made me appreciate central air and no crawling bugs or lizards.

I spent most of my life wondering where the next meal was going to come from. My parents spent nights without sleep worrying about the next house payment. Both of my parents worked in the fields picking or chopping cotton, and harvesting the season's fruits and vegetables. My mother also cleaned homes and ironed clothes for people on the weekends. My father also irri-gated farm lands day and night. He sang in the local bars during the weekends for extra money.

All family efforts went to support and educate four children. In the spring we migrated picking cotton as far as Texarkana, Texas, but returned to south Texas by September 1, so that the children would not miss any school. When I was thirteen years old, the family began to migrate to Chicago so that my father and sister could work in the local factories. The rest of the family picked cucumbers all week. On weekends I cleaned neighbors' homes and baby sat. When I became sixteen, I started to work in local factories during the summer. I worked part-time at a chicken processing market and also baby sat on the weekends. Eventually, three children graduated from high school, but my oldest sister was an eighth grade dropout. My brother has two years of college and my younger sister is a Spanish/English teacher.

In 1968, I became a licensed vocational nurse. I was very task oriented. In 1970, I graduated from Pan American College with an associate's degree in nursing and became a registered nurse. I was in charge of a Critical Care Unit. I enjoyed the emer-gency-save-a-life climate for about twelve years. Still, I was task-oriented. By this time, I was married with two young boys. Frustrated with myself and needing a higher level of accomplish-ment I graduated with a bachelor of science in nursing from UT at Arlington in l982. Now what ? My husband's retirement from the Air Force in 1982 influenced our return to South Texas. Again, I found myself in a task-oriented job. In 1985, I pursued and then graduated with a master of science in nursing administration from Corpus Christi State University.

After a year I realized that although I had the communica-tion and teaching skills for patient care, I did not have the polit-ical savvy to survive the work force . . . at least not at the level that I wanted. Feelings of being cheated by the educational sys-tem were a reality. I expected to cause an impact in health care with a master's degree but I was wrong. I felt I was not making a difference.

By 1994, when I defended my doctoral dissertation at the University of Houston, my level of frustration had decreased. My role at the job setting had also evolved. I learned that the obstacles and frustrations I experienced were mostly my own perceptions. It was how I perceived events and people. I finally learned to win wars and not battles. I became more focused on the important things in life—first, a Higher Being; second, family; and third, my job. When I accepted these priorities, I felt a greater level of satisfaction with myself. Listening, touching, patience, and understanding are now very central to my being a nurse. I wish I had had these qualities in 1970. What a great nurse I would have been!

In 1986, my mother's death impacted my life forever. In nursing and helping my mother die, I realized that death is natural and as important as life. Death is not the end of the world; it is only an event as natural as birth. Ten years after my mother's death my oldest sister told me I had the happiest look on my face the moment mother died. I explained how at the moment of her death, I saw this big Indian at the peak of a mountain with arms raised toward the sky who then became an eagle and flew away. I felt that it was mother's spirit separating from her body moving toward transcendance. The pain and suffering had closed and Mother was at peace.

Now, I am more empathetic and understanding with patients and people around me. I am not so critical. I do not see life being black and white. The gray area is a greater part of the picture . . . of life. I've learned that 10% of what happens to us in life is external and 90% is what comes from within the inner self.

Currently one of my responsibilities is to increase patient satisfaction by addressing patient/family complaints. Many of these involve the unwillingness to accept death of a loved one by the family. Many of our families do not understand the multisystem involvement as a result of diabetes and hypertension. When death occurs it is a surprise "because the only thing wrong was diabetes." Emotional support, empathy, and understanding need to be demonstrated by health care providers. In addressing these situations, such as education about diabetes, is a need in South Texas. I slowly, gently, and calmly explain the effects of diabetes which helps the family understand the impending death. I also explain that the health care providers did nothing to prompt the loved one's death. Knowledge and understanding of cultural differences has been an asset in my dealing with families whose loved one is dying. I believe Therapeutic Touch is one way to facilitate the transfer of inner, spiritual energy which helps sustain families during the death and grieving process.

Success, accomplishments, and happiness are a lifelong journey. In 1972, a Jewish physician friend of mine, Dr. Rottenstein, told me, "Patience and tolerance are a man's best assets." From Heaven I see him smiling at me because I guess he saw some of himself in me.

JoEllen Koerner
RN, PhD, FAAN

Senior Vice President of Patient Services, Sioux Valley Hospital, Sioux Falls, South Dakota

I was born in a small Mennonite community of 1,000 second generation immigrants who came to America seeking religious freedom. Half of my ancestors settled in a Mennonite colony along the river at the edge of town. My own great-grandparents chose to "live in the world, but not of the world." Translated into contemporary life, it created a living situation similar to the Amish and Quaker communities in this country. The community established its own schools which spoke only our German dialect. A strict code of ethics and dress separated these people from the neighboring communities.

Upon entering school at age six I began to experience the larger world. By this time, American ways had become commonplace among the non-Mennonites in the community. It was here that I began to learn the English language, a broader way of thinking and being that transcended the world view offered in my early childhood.

The women of my ancestry provided a profound influence in my life. My great-Grandmother, who had come from Russia at age five, was a slight woman garbed in a long black dress and delicately crocheted collar that was the dress code of the day. Her long white, never-cut hair was always neatly pulled into a bun on top of her tiny frame. Though she never had formal education, she was wise to the eyes of the initiated. Her storytelling was compelling. She would entertain me for hours with tales of other places and other times in a way that formed a deep sense of respect for diversity in my world view.

A legacy of strong and imaginative women was carried out by my paternal grandmother who was to be the most powerful influence in my life. This precious woman taught me the art of living simply where we are planted, living an ordinary life extremely well. She never ceased to display a deep sense of awe, wonder, and connection. Each experience was enacted as if for the first time, while always she extracted new mysteries hidden deeply in the familiar. In the 92 years of her life she never did run out of discoveries in her little corner of the universe! She showed me the difference between "having it all" and "having everything." Differentiating between needs and wants, she lived life in its simplest form. This simple approach to life was the ultimate exemplar of freedom! She challenged me to deal with what I was, where I was, and why I existed at all.

Though not a saint, grandmother walked through life with a barefoot soul; authentic, alert, aware, grateful, and only partially at home. Because of her influence I am currently taking off my socks.

I discovered in my shared experiences with grandmother that power comes from not having; that in scarcity lies abundance. When we are not surrounded or encumbered with "things" we have abundant space for authentic thought and creative action. Thus began my initiation into the paradox of living: when I stand alone I truly know community; when I am powerless, I can make my most powerful choices; the more I know the less I know; by standing in place I can see many realms; my life makes no difference while simultaneously it makes all the difference in the world. Paradox intertwines polar opposites so closely that the heart of one can be found in the other.

From my earliest memory, I wanted to be a nurse. I ran many animals through my first community-based nursing clinic. Stray cats and dogs, birds with injured wings, my sister's sprained ankle, and my brother's laceration from tangling with a broken bottle while wading the river were all tended with equal diligence. I found great joy in standing alongside those who are faced with physical challenges. Simultaneously, I was frequently sought out to "listen" to the problems and stories of others. I always told the individual I had no answers for them, and was amazed at how they always seemed to find the answer themselves just by laying things out to a listening ear.

I was fortunate that my desires matched the opportunities facing women of my era. We could choose between being a teacher, secretary, or a nurse. It also was a role highly valued by my Mennonite community. So upon graduation I found myself heading for Sioux Valley Hospital School of Nursing. This institution was my personal birthplace, my professional birthplace, and eventually the setting where I would live out most of my nursing career.

Mennonites believe that faith and action are inseparable, and voluntary service is an expectation. So the summer of high school graduation I went to Gulfport, Mississippi and worked in a youth camp. The group was a mixture of ages and races, and this was the summer the Civil Rights Bill was signed. We were exposed to bomb threats, kicked out of cafes, and barred from swimming in the ocean. The movie, "Mississippi Burning," has great personal meaning to me. It was in this setting that I learned that good things (like democracy) and well-intended people (like US citizens) hold a dark side driven by fear and ignorance. This experience planted a seed regarding the rights and abilities of each individual which I was able to honor by implementing shared governance with the nursing practice many years later.

I have lived a very common life and experienced abundance beyond measure. My career reflects that of so many others. I moved from staff nurse to the role of nurse manager. Taking three years off to raise twin babies, I returned to work for a rural clinic. I quickly became a physician's assistant (we had no access to nurse practitioner education in South Dakota at the time) and found myself carrying a case load in two rural communities. Shortly after that I was invited to teach, and ultimately administer a nursing program at Freeman Junior College. This led to an appointment on the South Dakota State Board of Nursing in the role of education consultant. I learned a great deal about both regulation and the variety of ways that people can learn in a rural sparsely populated state. The creativity of the various programs never ceased to amaze and delight me.

Suddenly, I found myself the executive director of the board and the administrative and political aspects of my life became highly developed. In this role I discovered that my Mennonite background, which encourages women to work through men, made me well suited to work with a primarily male legislature. It was also this position that created an invitation from Sioux Valley Hospital to return to the place of my birth as the nursing vice president. I turned down the offer three times telling the recruiter "I know what I don't know, and I don't know how to run large organizations"! The wonderful woman inviting me to the position said, "Know the difference between inability and inexperience. You have not done this work before, but you have acquired the skills for it in your past work." It was one of the most profound pieces of advice given to me on this journey towards mastery.

I have had the privilege of walking alongside this extraordinary nursing practice for thirteen years. They have taught me so many valuable lessons. In nursing we are taught to minister to the individual and the family, and our lens is primarily about the patient. I have learned that groups come together as a multicellular organism. There is a collective group culture, group values, group world view. There is a shared context in which we function. Just as we develop strategies for patients and families, some nurses are called to develop strategies for collectives and aggregate groups. I believe that health care reform will take this model of caring and healing to communities, and specific patient populations as well.

In leading and following a nursing practice, I believe that nurse executives offer several things, just as staff nurses offer these to patients. We provide a vision of what is possible so that others can go beyond where they are in the moment. We offer energy when they have little because of multiple demands on their time, wisdom, and compassion. We become a support so they can venture where they have never been before, knowing that we will stop them if they go too far afield. We celebrate their creations because they are life-giving. We embrace their failures because they are a demonstration of courage and commitment to what could be. We weep with their disappointments because we share a spirit of tenderness. We experience hope because we are a community of caregivers, caring for a community of humans who share our core essence. Mostly, we give and receive love, the only element that can truly heal.

Standing alongside someone in that sacred space of suffering, or in the transformational moments of life or death, is a great privilege. We are invited into this space because society needs us. When we enter this sacred ground we must honor our social accountability to the people we are privileged to serve. This calls us to uphold the values and principles of healing in this time of health care reform. Nursing must be the moral force that will maintain the focus on actions and outcomes that honor life. In this way society will move towards the self-actualization which is their birthright, and part of our human legacy. It is a privilege to be part of nursing—a powerful force for healing in a chaotic and changing world.

Jean Marie Umlor
RSM, RN, MNA, HNC

*Coordinator of Holistic Clinical Practice,
Mercy Health Services North,
Grayling, Michigan*

I remember the moment as if it was yesterday. I was in the third grade at our little rural Catholic school. Each school day began with the Latin Mass. We didn't understand the words but the rituals attracted even a third grader's imagination! As we left the Church that morning I looked up to the gallery and one of the girls from our parish, now a student nurse at the nearby Catholic Hospital, was there. I remember saying, "Someday I'm going to be a nurse!"

The past fifty years has been my journey as a nurse; a woman's journey of facing her own healing, a woman searching for healing connections with other women, a woman seeking to be a healing presence among the sick-poor, a woman seeking to change the systems that keep people sick and poor, a woman celebrating healing.

The seeds of this inspiration had its beginning with my farm family of German-Dutch descent in a small town called Conklin, Michigan. I am the middle child of seven children, born in 1936 at a time when resources were very limited. However, we had a farm, a loving mom and dad, and we learned that family, work, family prayer, family fun, and family support were integral to our life on the farm.

As a middle child, I soon learned how to negotiate my way through the family interactions, grade school, high school, and into the School of Nursing at St. Mary's Hospital, Grand Rapids, Michigan. It was a three-year program recently reorganized into a twenty-seven month program with an optional nine month internship program. I was the first of the Umlor family to leave home, go thirty miles away, and live in a dorm for education beyond high school. In retrospect, for a middle child, this was the easiest part. The personal pattern in the weaving of my living was emerging.

The image of weaving has a particular significance for me because I am a weaver. I have learned to value the source of the material from a living being and the ongoing preparation of the material which includes the cutting, washing, shaping, pulling, and spinning of the material. I know the effort it takes to measure the material and prepare it for the loom. I have experienced the delight of seeing a pattern emerge when I carefully notice how I, the loom, and the material work together. I have felt the effort it takes to re-weave a section that was not according to a pattern. I have felt the comfort of the sweater or blanket for many weeks after all the initial effort. I have enjoyed the beauty of the blanket with many others.

The patterns of my life as a nurse have the same features of creation. The fabric is from a rich, living family life that opened to me a desire to be a nurse. The materials of myself as a young woman were prepared; it was washed, stretched, cleansed, and pulled through my early education as a nurse and my entrance into the Community of the Sisters of Mercy, Detroit, Michigan. So many persons were the gentle-women who helped me through these early years as a nurse and as a Sister of Mercy. These women and the many events of my living took on a pattern that continues to be revealed. Some of these include the experience of being a nursing supervisor when I hardly knew how to be a nurse; the joy of new life for religious women in the Catholic Church following the Vatican II event; the opportunity to gain knowledge through a Master's Degree in Nursing Service Administration from the University of Iowa and a Master's Degree in Christian Spirituality

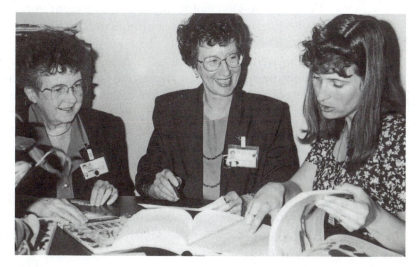

from Creighton University, Omaha, Nebraska; being a nurse administrator during the beginnings of primary nursing, critical care units, and trauma centers; working as an outreach nurse practitioner in the inner city of Detroit; sharing nursing knowledge with the nurses in the Island of Palau and the Marshall Island; starting a home care program in rural northern Michigan; initiating the Parish Nurse in Michigan; and working as an outreach worker in a domestic violence shelter for women and children.

The weaving is incomplete without the contrasting threads, the shadow side of my own person, of the nursing profession; of my religious community and of the various communities in which I worked. I had to learn to notice, to embrace, and to integrate the painful times of my living: the insecurity in my own person and the belief system that my worth was my work; the loss of nursing as a home; the loss of my Church as a home; the loss of my friends who choose to leave the Sisters of Mercy; the rapid changes in health care; all my dissatisfaction with the sick-care system; the disillusion with so many systems and structures. All that I had valued was disintregating and I was not sure if life had any meaning. In the midst of this journey of the weaving, I discovered so many companions who shared the journey with me. We began to connect, to remember, and to share our story as women, healers, lovers, and as persons concerned with other women and children and our earth. Our connection in a deep level of spirituality was a key aspect of the pattern that emerged among us.

I began to re-identify my own personal pattern as a wounded healer who journeyed with other women and men in the healing of others. The members of the American Holistic Nurses' Association and the Holistic Nurse Certificate Program were some of my new partners. Rich patterns of life were shown to me through all of my living as a woman, a nurse, a healer; as a person concerned with health, healing, spirituality, ecology, feminism, politics; as a member of a faith community called Sisters of Mercy.

At this point in my life, I feel wrapped in the comfort of nursing as a healer who knows the wounds, the pain, and the birth of new life. I share the beauty of who I and nursing are becoming as healers for each other, for women and children, for our earth, and for the ongoing creation and revelation of a healing and loving presence I call God—the Master Weaver or the Goddess Weaver!

Bonnie Wesorick
RN, MS

*Director, Clinical Practice
Model (CPM) Resource Center,
Butterworth Hospital,
Grand Rapids, Michigan*

The invitation to write about my personal journey as a nurse healer evoked many feelings within me. I found myself wondering about the importance of one person's story. What is relevant or most important is that the stories of nurse healers be captured—not because nurses are the largest group of health care providers in the world, but because of the nature of their work. Nurses are intimately present during so many vulnerable and special moments across the life span, including birthing-birth, living-life, deathing-death. With this privilege comes a wisdom and an accountability to speak to that wisdom, especially during these changing, chaotic times of great transformation within the health care system. The insight and understanding of the importance to tell the stories of nurse healers is a cause for celebration. It was this realization that caused me to feel honored and humbled to have been asked to share my story.

There is no specific beginning to my journey as a nurse healer. There is no one event that led to my choice to become a nurse. It seems, but only as I look back, that it was a natural evolution of my life's relationships. My roots have been nourished by a hard working, middle-class family where the focus was on each other and family. My strong Judeo-Christian roots, both in home and school, reinforced my view that life is a gift; I am free; purpose and meaning in life is in relationships, and I have many choices and will be held accountable for my choices.

In looking back, I was not totally sensitive to or aware of two factors that influenced my choice to be a nurse. One was the status of women during the late fifties and early sixties, and the second was the financial feasibility of continued education because of my family's fiscal status. The image of women in nursing and the inexpensive diploma school both enhanced my choice. With little access to academic advisors who often explain test and class performance, I was not stimulated by multiple options often provided to students today. Had that been the case, my strong math skills may have led me to be an engineer—a scary thought!

I have always been surrounded by love, laughter, hard work, and fun which allowed me to become a dreamer, a risk taker, strong, willful, sometimes labeled as a naive idealist, and an optimist. I believe that because of my family life and other life relationships, I was driven by a desire to contribute, to love, and to reach my personal potential. Nursing was in synchrony with my personal mission.

The experience of a diploma school of nursing both strengthened and inhibited what I would come to know as the work of healing. The relationships with patients and classmates strengthened my learning. The rituals, patterns, teaching methods, and routines inhibited my learning. The step from a hospital-based school of nursing to the hospital setting as new practitioner was natural. It is the reality of hospital practice that explains my personal evolution as nurse healer.

I am from the first generation of nurses to experience technology in the practice field. I personally believe that this timing not only impacted my practice evolution, but also every nurse's evolution who practiced in the hospital. In the sixties I remember standing with the family at the bedside of a person dying. I was acutely aware of the grief and wondered why we could not do more to help the person live. Knowing that a person's spirit will leave a body that cannot sustain life created in me a strong and natural focus on how to strengthen the body so to sustain life.

I got caught up in the excitement of technological advancement that helped us keep people alive. I became immersed in the work of medicine. Insidiously, my focus left nursing and centered on medicine. My art and science of medicine grew every day with immense rewards. I was moved by the wisdom of Florence Nightingale who, over one hundred years ago, said, "Experience teaches me that nursing and medicine must never be mixed up, it spoils both." My art and science of nursing became blurred, challenged, and devalued by myself and a busy, expanding medically focused team. There soon became little time to nurse, but look what inroads were being made!

Then, as I stood with the family by the side of their loved one who was almost miraculously living, not dying, I was acutely aware of the human response of the patient and family—the grief, the pain, the response that no technology, no pill, no tasks, no treatment could help. My relationships with them helped me understand the importance of the choice I had made to nurse. Hope for them related to my ability to nurse, not how good I was at medicine. It was this realization that ignited my soul and created a strong desire to nurse.

That desire was soon challenged. First, it was my weakness in nursing's unique art and science. It had not advanced in the same proportion as my understanding of medicine. Secondly, I would learn that my lack of nursing knowledge would pale in the face of a greater reality. The second reality was the practice culture surrounding me and thousands of other practitioners. The culture was designed and structured to enhance the practice of medicine, not nursing. Good nursing meant supporting good medicine. Some normalities became glaring barriers. The whole culture evolved around medical diagnosis, disease, body parts, doctors' orders, policies, and procedures. The environment was one of hierarchical relationships and boss/subordinate, not partnerships in health care. I wondered how and when it happened and what could be done. I decided to do something about it. It is this sec-

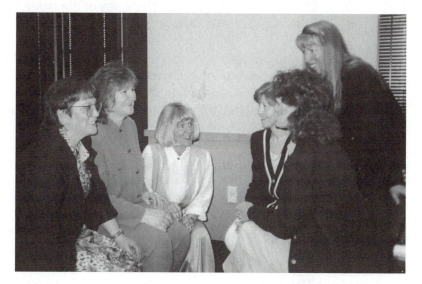

ond challenge that would lead to my real work as healer and probably led me to be asked to share my story.

I began to speak about the essence of nursing and the need to create an empowered, healing professional practice environment. I soon learned I was not alone. I was surrounded by thousands of colleagues practicing in hospital settings who longed to nurse but no longer dared to hope it would become a reality. I was driven by the passion, the personal stories of nursing care told to me by colleagues. It was from these relationships and the dialogue with colleagues that my clarity on the essence of nursing emerged. The formation of partnerships with nurses gave me direction and helped me understand the importance and necessity of creating environments to support nurses to practice our unique profession. I realized if I cared about patients, I must first care about the nurses giving the care. My work is about healing the healers.

At the time I began my work, the majority of all nurses practiced in the fast-paced hospital setting. In the business of the setting, we disconnected from one another in our choice—our beautiful, important choice to nurse. This resulted in our collective understanding of the essence of nursing being lost in the institutional rituals, tasks, policies, and procedures of the clinical settings. As colleagues we seldom talked about our practice or our relationships as healers. Our conversations evolved around tasks to be done. The words of Thomas Merton warn of the danger of such reality when he said, "To live in communion, in genuine dialogue with others, is absolutely necessary if man is to remain human. But to live in the midst of others sharing nothing with them but the common noise and the general distraction, isolates a man in the worst way, separates him from reality in a way that is almost painless. It divides him off and separates him from other men and from his true self." The focus on tasks and the rituals, or the noise of the day, painlessly divided us off from our relationships as healers both with each other, and with the people we are privileged to give care.

With the feedback, wisdom, and energy of thousands of nurses, I have initiated and implemented a framework to create an empowered, healing practice environment. The principle-driven, systems thinking framework supports the practitioners in their transition from a medical, institutional, and hierarchical practice to one focused on health, the essence of nursing and partnerships.

It is being used in over thirty-three rural, community, and university settings in seventeen states and two countries. In order to continue this important work, the Clinical Practice Model Resource Center has been founded at Butterworth Hospital, Grand Rapids, Michigan. The mission of the center is to establish partnerships and world linkages for the generation of collective knowledge and wisdom that continually improves the structure, process, and outcomes of professional practice and community health care services. The work is driven by core beliefs that speak to the essence of our mission and vision as healers.

Although uncertain who spoke the following words, they eloquently speak to the sacredness of our work: "Our deeds are like stones cast into the pool of time, although they themselves may disappear, their ripples extend to eternity." My greatest learning on this journey is that to be a nurse healer one must first heal the self. It is then that the ripples of our work will nourish the roots of this humanity.

Part

4

THE
HEALING
JOURNEY

Chapter

8 | THE HEALING JOURNEY

THE EVOLVING PROCESS

Becoming a nurse healer is an evolving process of integrating the art and science of caring and healing. It is an extraordinary, rewarding, and fulfilling experience. As we learn about the dynamics of healing, we have more opportunities to live healthy and inspired lives. This healing journey into the exploration of the unity and relatedness of all aspects of living and dying awakens the healing potentials within self and others. Ask yourself four significant questions:

1. What do you know about the meaning of healing?
2. What can you do each day to facilitate healing in yourself?
3. What is the essence of being a nurse healer?
4. What can you do to enhance your qualities of being a nurse healer?

INTEGRATION OF HEALING RITUALS

Healing rituals and the exploration of the creative arts are a way of connecting with the sacred life force. Rituals allow for a non-interfering attention of being present in the moment that allows natural healing to flow. As we explore rituals and the creative arts, we can evoke presence and inner peace. Healing rituals provide special sacred and quality time that empowers us to transfer this experience to clinical practice as well as to all areas of our lives.

Healing rituals are essential in the caring-healing process. Our anxiety, worries, and fears are reduced. As we learn how to integrate healing rituals into our lives, we can better assist clients to lessen their anxieties, worries, and fears. We are better able to assist them to deal with their feelings of helplessness or to deal with crisis, trauma, procedures, pain, and daily events. Some rituals for clinical practice may be the way we hold a client's hand with intention to be present in the moment; the active listening to a family member; to take rhythmic deep breaths to be in the present moment; or the use of a prayer or affirmation. We must first know how to incorporate healing rituals in our daily lives before we can successfully teach others how to use them in their own lives.

An important aspect of inner work in our fast-paced lives is to create a time for rituals that have specific meaning. For example, what are your healing rituals that assist you in being present in the moment? What do you do when clients and their families are faced with symptoms or tests, or are confronted with decisions about medical or surgical intervention or end-of-life decisions? What healing rituals do you share with clients and families to assist them as they make their decisions? We must always remember that we can never make a decision for others, but we can introduce them to ways to create a space of recognizing their inner wisdom that resides within them. The ritual guide for getting well, as seen in Table 8-1, is excellent for guiding clients and families with rituals and decision-making. We can also use these guidelines when we or our family members are faced with similar situations.

In creating a ritual, there are no absolute rules that should be followed. A few guidelines are that a ritual should have a structure—a beginning, a middle, and an end. It helps to plan the details carefully in advance, such as what you do in anticipation of a special house guest. You give attention to details in a guest room by adding fresh flowers and books of art or poetry at a bedside, etc., so that a sacred space is created. This also happens when we create a sacred space to be alone and reflect on healing awareness. We deepen our understanding of being connected with self, others, and a Higher Self. This special time is what helps us with healing our own lives so that we are available for others.

TABLE 8-1 *The First Ritual Guide to Getting Well.*

This ritual helps you decide what to do if you are diagnosed with the unknowable, the unthinkable, the awful, or the so-called incurable. By doing this, you can better determine how to survive treatment, yourself, your friends and family, and life in general.

1. Find a quiet place, a healing place, and go there. This might be a corner of your favorite room where you have placed gifts, pictures, a candle, or other symbols that signal peace and inner reflections to you. Or it might be in a park, under an old tree, or in a special place known for its spirit, such as high on a sacred mountain or on the cliffs overlooking a coastline or in the quiet magnificence of a forest.

2. Ask questions of your inner self about what your diagnosis or treatment means in your life. How will life change? What are your resources, your strengths, your reasons for staying alive? These deeply philosophical or spiritual issues often come to mind when problems are diagnosed. Listen with as quiet a mind as possible for any answers or messages that come from within, or from your higher source of guidance.

3. Take this time, knowing that very few problems advance so quickly that you must rush into making decisions about them immediately, without first gaining some perspective.

4. Find at least one friend or advocate who can be leveled-headed when you think you are going crazy; who can be positive for you when you are absolutely certain you are doomed; who can listen when your head is buzzing with uncertainty.

5. Love yourself. Ask yourself moment by moment whether what surrounds you is nurturing and life-giving. If the answer is no, back off from it. Kindly tell all negative-thinking people that you will not be seeing them while you are going through this. You may need never to see them again, and this is your right and obligation to yourself.

6. Assess your belief system. What do you believe? How did you get to believe it in the first place? What is really happening inside you and outside you? How serious is it? What will it take to get you well?

7. Gather information, keeping an open mind. Everyone who offers to treat you or give you advice has their lives invested in what they tell you. Stand back and listen thoughtfully.

8. Now go and hire your healing team. Remember, you hired them—you can fire them. They are in the business of performing a service for you, and you are paying their salaries. Sometimes this relationship gets confused. Make sure they are talking to each other. You are in command. You are the captain of the healing team.

9. Don't let anyone talk you into treatment you don't believe in or don't understand. Keep asking questions. Replace anyone who acts too busy to answer your qustions. Chances are, they're also too busy to do their best work for you.

TABLE 8-1 *Continued.*

10. Don't agree on any diagnostic or lab tests unless someone you trust can give you good reasons why they are being ordered. If the tests are not going to change your treatment, they are an expensive and dangerous waste of your time.

11. Sing your own song, write your own story, take your own spiritual journey through a journal or diary. A threat to health and well-being can be a trigger to becoming and doing all those things you've been putting off for the "right" time.

12. Consider these maxims in your journey:
    • Everything cures somebody, and nothing cures everybody.
    • There are no simple answers to complex issues, like why people get sick in the first place.
    • Sometimes disease is inexplicable to mortal minds.

13. You will not be intimidated by the overbearing world of medicine or alternative health know-it-alls but can thoughtfully take the best from several worlds.

14. You can teach gentleness and compassion to the most arrogant doctor and the crankiest nurse. Tell them that you need your mind and soul nurtured, as well as the best medical treatment possible in order to get well. If they are not up to it, you'll find someone someplace who is.

Source: Reprinted from *Rituals of Healing: Using Imagery for Health and Wellness* by J. Achterberg, B. Dossey, and L. Kolkmeier, pp. 32–33. Bantam Books, 1994. Reprinted by permission of J. Achterberg, B. Dossey, and L. Kolkmeier, copyright 1994.

As we begin the first phase of a ritual, the separation phase, it is a symbolic act of breaking away from life's busy activities. For example, it might involve going to a quiet room for fifteen to twenty minutes, and taking shoes off, sitting on a pillow on the floor, putting on the answering machine, and honoring the silence. As we go to this sacred healing place, we might sacralize the space with a special object such as a burning candle or focus on a healing image that brings a sense of calmness.

As we enter the second phase of ritual, the transition phase, we can more easily identify areas in our life that need attention. It is a time of facing the shadow, the hero's journey, where we recognize the dark, the difficult, as we reflect on what is real and worthy and in need of healing in the deepest sense. It is the time to go into an unknown terrain, the *limen*, the meaning threshold, where we leave one way of being to enter into another way of participating.

Finally we enter the last phase of the ritual, the return phase, where we reenter into real life. This phase allows for a formal release, putting aside or leaving old patterns of fears, anger, or memories that no longer serve us. We are challenged to integrate a new way of acting, choosing, and relating, to "walk our talk" of healing awareness.

Healing awareness is our ability to discipline ourselves to be present in the moment and understand the meaning of the moment. What surfaces with this state of being present in the moment is a noninterfering attention that allows natural healing to flow. One way to become more aware of being mindful is through a mindfulness practice.

MINDFULNESS PRACTICE

A mindfulness practice is a wonderful opportunity to learn how to be present in the moment with our body, mind, and spirit. Healing happens in the present moment, not in the past or in the future. As we set aside time each day to practice mindfulness, we learn to recognize essential steps for healing. These are such qualities as softening, opening, receiving, forgiving, empathy, compassion, truth, and loving kindness.

There are many ways to begin your practice. You might use strategies such as relaxation, imagery, music, prayer, meditation, or a meditative movement practice such as walking meditation, yoga or Tai'Chi. Some guidelines for beginning a mindfulness practice are:

- Set aside time each day to develop a practice of sitting mindfully (or mindfulness movement) for a minimum of ten minutes each day.

- Find a quiet, comfortable place to practice.

- If your mind wanders and begins to attend to things that need to be done, places to go, unfinished business, or conversations with self or others, bring your mind back to the present moment. Some ways to do this are to focus on the breath, just watching the in and out breath. You may wish to see each thought as it comes. In your mind you may wish to place each thought on a leaf and see it flowing away in a stream of water.

You might find that you get bored with practice, cut it short, get uncomfortable, get angry, dislike certain emotions, or decide that nothing is happening. These are natural events as we learn to quiet the constant mind chatter or self-talk. Just approach your practice with a sense of exploring, opening, and lightening to the experience of being in the moment. Let go of any competitiveness or thinking there is a right way. If any uncomfortable emotions or memories come forward, you can either be with them for new insight or take a deep breath, open your eyes, and these experiences leave. If you wish to delve into these uncomfortable emotions and feel stuck, you may wish to seek professional assistance from a nurse therapist or a counselor who specializes in certain areas, for example, abuse work, loss/grief work, etc.

As we learn to be in the moment, we access our natural wisdom. This occurs because we begin to notice the nature of our body, mind, and spirit as we create a state of intention and presence, recognizing new understanding and inner peace.

JOURNALING

Another way to become more open to healing is through journaling. This is a special process of recording events, thoughts, feelings, dreams, fears, losses, trauma/wounds, healing moments, and inner and external healing resources. There is not a correct or right way to journal. To gain a deeper understanding of the journaling process and self-reflection you may find that your journaling may go from structured to free-form without structure. A few suggestions are offered:

- Set aside a minimum of five minutes a day to record in your journal.
- Find a quiet, comfortable place to journal.
- Use different tools to enhance your creativity such as music, relaxation, and imagery exercises prior to journaling.

- Choose a special notebook for journaling. You might also find that you prefer to write on a loose piece of blank or lined paper and keep these pages in a folder.

- Select a writing pen or colored markers to record words and images. This often allows your recorded words and images to take on a deeper significance.

EXPLORING CREATIVITY

A healing environment allows creativity to flow. Personal preference determines how we each create our healing environment. Some items might include floor pillows for your experiential exercises, colorful posters, flowers, plants, and running water that flows into a small open reservoir vase or container (small, inexpensive pump and container can be found at a garden nursery). You may want to find a place in nature for walking or meditations where you can be tuned into the natural rhythms and cycles of nature. These naturally occurring events in nature can serve as metaphors (the changing of the seasons, planting seeds, flowering, going into hibernation, etc.) and can remind us of the natural rhythms of our lives as well.

Many art objects and supplies can be integrated into our healing rituals. These include the imagination, candles, music, drums, altar or sacred space, circle, masks, songs, incense, healing symbols, totems, fetishes, poetry, chants, feathers, colored yarns, crayons, colored construction paper, pictures, stories, talking stick, flowers, water, earth elements, clay, and other art supplies. It is most helpful to gather these art supplies and various healing objects in one place. You might find it most useful to place these supplies in baskets to be easily transported from one place to another or to be stored.

Find your own personal style. Use different techniques and complementary modalities that allow your passion for caring and healing to emerge. Use your creative gifts. Which arts speak to you? How do you respond to music, art, paintings, weaving, sculpting, etc. If you are not comfortable with your artistic side, you might find a mentor or coach. Discover professionals and other healers in your community who integrate different healing modalities in their practices. Take the time to experience these individuals through private sessions, workshops, or public lectures.

SHARING OUR HEALING STORIES

An important part of the evolving process of developing as a nurse healer is to be able to share our personal story such as we read about in Part 3. Nurse healers are aware that through sharing circles and time to be in dialogue with colleagues, true healing occurs. Personal sharing allows us time to focus on the essential steps in healing, presence, the art of guiding, and real versus pseudo-listening. Sharing circles can be 15 to 20 minutes or longer in groups of 3 to 6 or more. These sharing circles provide opportunities to exchange healing moments and any personal aspects that are in need of healing. This is to encourage the "listening council process."

There are only a few special guidelines. When we are mindful of the dialogue process and active listening, we can speak "from our heart." When the skills of speaking with intention are developed, an individual is able to be present and avoid superficial comments. To encourage reflection, a moment of silence before sharing is helpful. This is not time for "psychoanalyzing" each other, but a time to practice presence in the moment and speaking from a place of authentic sharing. This helps in keeping the dialogue open because we learn to build trust and concern for self and others.

A talking stick or healing object may be used by a person before talking. Before speaking, a person will pick up a talking stick or a healing object and speak with intention. Only the person holding the talking stick or healing object speaks. As we learn to be present with self, to hear stories of healing, joy, or deep pain, and to share the struggles and triumphs of one's own journey with others, we learn to validate the importance of caring and healing moments. This is a time to come with an openness to develop new skills, to actively participate. We increase our understanding of what is meant by "allowing healing presence into each moment of nursing."

BROWN BAG LUNCH SESSIONS

The question is often asked how to transfer these ideas into mainstream nursing. A useful strategy is in classroom presentation style. It is best done off of a busy care unit so that nurses can listen and share and be without patient responsibilities.

For example, two colleagues might post a note that announces a certain date each month for a brown bag lunch session. The note might give a few ideas about the purpose of the gathering such as to explore ways to enhance caring and healing in clinical practice.

Prior to the session, it is helpful to develop, plan, and prepare a handout on the topic chosen that includes a few recent articles and research from various resources. A case study and an experiential session related to the topic may also be helpful to reinforce and integrate the learning. Further brown bag lunch sessions might include a guest speaker who uses different alternative/complementary modalities, self-assessment tools to use in clinical practice, and other colleagues invited to share their areas of expertise.

As we develop our healing potentials and deepen our understanding of presence and healing, learning how to "walk the talk" of holism, we will be role models for professional practice and daily living. To nurture our body, mind, and spirit we must continue to integrate cognitive knowledge as well as intuition and creativity. This leads to sharing and healing of self and how to integrate these dimensions in all aspects of one's being. This evolving process builds trust in self as well as how to create a healing community with colleagues. When we do this we can shape the profession to arrive on the doorsteps of the twenty-first century as nurse healers who practice the "finest of the fine art and science of nursing."

R E F E R E N C E S

Achterberg, J., Dossey, B. M., & Kolkmeier, L. (1994). *Rituals of healing*. New York: Bantam Books.

Dossey, B. M. (ed). (1997). *American Holistic Nurses' Association Core Curriculum for Holistic Nursing*. Gaithersburg, MD: Aspen Publishers, Inc.

Dossey, B. M., Keegan, L., Guzzetta, C., & Kolkmeier, L. (1995). *Holistic nursing: A handbook for practice*, (2nd ed.). Gaithersburg, MD: Aspen Publishers, Inc.

Dossey, B. M., Keegan, L., Guzzetta, C. E., & Kolkmeier, L. (1995). *Instructor's manual for holistic nursing: A handbook for practice*. (2nd ed.). Gaithersburg, MD: Aspen Publishers, Inc.

Dossey, B. M., Keegan, L., & Guzzetta, C. E. (1995). *The art of caring: Holistic healing using relaxation, imagery, music therapy and touch*. Boulder, CO: Sounds True.

Frisch, N. C., & Kelley, J. (1996). *Healing life's crises: A guide for nurses*. Albany, NY: Delmar Publishers.

Hover-Kramer, D. (1996). *Healing touch: A resource for health care professionals*. Albany, NY: Delmar Publishers.

Hover-Kramer, D. & Shames, K. H. (1997). *Energetic approaches to emotional healing*. Albany, NY: Delmar Publishers.

Journal of Holistic Nursing Practice. (1997). (The official publication of the American Holistic Nurses' Association). Thousand Oakes, CA: Sage Periodicals Press.

Keegan, L. (1994). *Nurse as healer*. Albany, NY: Delmar Publishers.

Olsen, M. (1997). *Healing the Dying*. Albany, NY: Delmar Publishers.

Rew, L. (1996). *Awareness in healing.* Albany, NY: Delmar Publishers.

Schaub, B. & Schaub, R. (1997). *Healing addictions.* Albany, NY: Delmar Publishers.

Shames, K. H. (1996). *Creative imagery in nursing.* Albany, NY: Delmar Publishers.

A P P E N D I X

RESOURCES

Organizations

American Holistic Nurses' Association (AHNA)
4101 Lake Boone Trail, Suite #201
Raleigh, North Carolina 27607
Phone   (919)787-5181
          (800) 278-AHNA
Fax   (919) 787-4916

*For information on the AHNA Certificate Program in Holistic Nursing, AHNCC Certification in Holistic Nursing, Interactive Guided Imagery, and related programs contact AHNA at above address.

Videos and Audiocassettes

Holistic Nursing

Contact: American Holistic Nurses' Association (AHNA)
           See address above

At the Heart of Healing: Experiencing Holistic Nursing

Contact: Kineholistic Foundation
           P.O. Box 719
           Woodstock, New York 12498
           (800) 255-1914, ext. 277

A Conversation on Caring with Jean Watson and Janet Quinn

Contact: National League for Nursing Press
            350 Hudson Street
            New York, New York 10014

Therapeutic Touch: Video Course for Healthcare Professionals (by Janet Quinn). Three tape set and Study Guide.

Contact: Haelan Works
            3080 3rd Street
            Boulder, Colorado 80304
            Phone/Fax: (303) 449-5790

Therapeutic Touch: A Home Study Video Course for Family Caregivers (by Janet Quinn). Produced by National League for Nursing Press.

Contact: Haelan Works
            3080 3rd Street
            Boulder, Colorado 80304
            Phone/Fax: (303) 449-5790

The Art of Caring (by Barbara M. Dossey, Lynn Keegan, and Cathie E. Guzzetta), Four audiocassette tape set and Study Guide.

Contact: Sounds True
            413 S. Arthur Ave.
            Louisville, Colorado 80027
            (800) 333-9185

Internet

Contact: http://www.ahna.org
            American Holistic Nurses' Association homepage

Contact: http://www.healthy.net
            For abundant healthcare information from Health
            World Online

G L O S S A R Y

Allopathic. The method of combating disease with techniques that produce effects different from those produced by the disease.

Alternative/complementary therapies. Interventions that focus on body-mind-spirit integration that evoke healing by an individual, between two individuals, or healing at a distance (relaxation, imagery, biofeedback, prayer, psychic healing, etc.); may be used as complements to conventional medical treatments.

Bio-psycho-social-spiritual. The major elements that give meaning to a person's existence.

Centering. Fine tuning of sensitivity to life's inner and outer patterns and processes; recognizing a state of balance of self and allowing the process of intuition to unfold.

Guide. One who helps others discover and recognize insights and healing awareness about their life journey.

Healing. A process of bringing parts of oneself together at a deep level of inner knowledge leading toward an integration and balance, with each part having equal importance and value; may also be referred to as self-healing or wholeness.

Holism. The view that an integrated whole has a reality independent of and greater than the sum of its parts.

Intention. Allowing the natural universal life force to flow and to experience inner calm and peace so that one's work may involve patterns of knowing and unknowing.

Intuition. Perceived knowing of things and events without the conscious use of rational processes.

Nurse healer. One who facilitates another person's growth and life processes toward wholeness (body-mind-spirit) or who assists with recovery from illness or with transition to peaceful death.

Presence. A state achieved when one moves within oneself to an inner reference of stability of being in the moment; a mode of "being with" rather than "doing to."

Polarities. The contrast of opposite qualities or states such as health and illness, birth and death.

Process. The continual changing and evolution of one's self through life; the reflection of meaning and purpose in living.

Relationships (healthy). One, two, or more nonjudgmental people with whom you share your interests, successes, and failures; people who facilitate and accelerate one's life potentials.

Spirituality. A broad concept that encompasses values, meaning, and purpose; one turns inward to the human traits of honesty, love, caring, wisdom, imagination, and compassion; existence of a quality of a higher authority, guiding spirit, or transcendence that is mystical; a flowing dynamic balance that allows and creates healing of body-mind-spirit; may or may not involve organized religion.

Transpersonal. Referring to experiences and meaning that go beyond individual and personal uniqueness; a unification with universal principles.

Transpersonal self. The sense of self that goes beyond the ego and "I" that does not identify itself as a single isolated individual; includes purpose, meaning, and values.

Wounded healer. Concept derived from Greek mythology, specifically the myth of Chiron, which suggests that even the greatest healers have inherent weaknesses and fallibility that should be recognized by the healer.

INDEX